Nailing The Medical School Interview:

A Harvard MD's Comprehensive Preparation Strategy

The prices and rates stated in this book are subject to change.
Library of Congress Control Number: 2015905168
ISBN: 978-1-936633-11-1
Edited by Sharon Miller
Cover design by Ali Raza
Interior layout by Booknook.Biz

Dedication

For Sharon Miller – sounding board,
teacher, and editor extraordinaire

Also by Dr. Suzanne M. Miller

The Medical School Admissions Guide:
A Harvard MD's Week-by-Week Admissions Handbook, 3ʳᵈ Ed

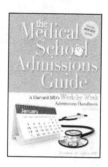

How to be Pre-Med:
A Harvard MD's Medical School Preparation Guide for Students and Parents

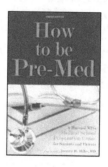

How to Get Into Medical School with a Low GPA (e-book)

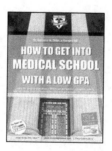

Table of Contents

Preface

Congratulations! If you are reading this book, it is likely you have been granted a medical school interview or expect to receive one soon. Given that 100% of US medical schools require an interview for admissions, obtaining an interview invite is a huge step forward in the admissions process. In fact, after completing your primary and secondary applications, it's the last step required to gain acceptance. And, according to a survey of medical school admissions committees conducted by the American Association of Medical Colleges (AAMC), interviews are the most important factor used to decide which applicants gain acceptance (Dunleavy DM). *The most important factor!* Fortunately, interview techniques can be learned and (when practiced) improved. So there is hope for all pre-meds who get to the interview stage.

Before we dive into the meat of medical school interview preparation, let me tell you a bit about myself and how I came to write this book. I started out as a driven and admittedly anxious pre-med trying to survive the competition at Harvard. Fortunately, through picking a well-suited major, falling into a crowd of brilliant and fun fellow pre-meds more interested in learning than competing, and having access to exceptional pre-med advisors, I excelled as an undergrad and landed a spot at Harvard Medical School. While in medical school, I gained the coveted position of Eliot House

Pre-Medical Committee co-chair, where I specialized in getting Harvard pre-meds into medical school and took a particular interest in interview preparation. Having learned the ins and outs of the admissions process, I then ventured out to Stanford for emergency medicine residency and began MDadmit, a medical admissions consultancy. Over a decade later, MDadmit has blossomed into a leading medical admissions company while I continue to teach and work clinically both in the US and abroad.

One of my main motivations for running MDadmit is to pay forward the help I received as a pre-med because I know access to excellent pre-med advisors is not universal. Further, I understand many pre-meds don't have the funds to hire admissions consultants. Thus, I decided to put the expert advice I offer my clients down on paper so that all pre-meds have access. This started with *The Medical School Admissions Guide* and continued with *How to Be Pre-Med* and *How to Get Into Medical School with a Low GPA*. During MDadmit mock interviews, clients kept asking why I hadn't written a book specifically directed at interview preparation. Though I discuss interviews in *The Medical School Admissions Guide*, I realized these clients had a great idea. The topic of medical school interviews deserves its own book. I certainly could have used an interview preparation guide as a pre-med, particularly one focusing on the most common and difficult questions and how to develop answers to them. Thus, *Nailing the Medical School Interview* was born. I do hope you find it improves your interview skills and increases your chances of medical school acceptance.

How to Use This Book

Medical school interviews can be daunting, given the sheer number of possible questions and the importance of what is at stake. But as you will see in this book, the questions can be broken into different categories to make them more approachable. Yet, even with the help of this categorization strategy, preparing thoroughly for a medical school interview takes time. I think the best time to prepare for interviews is after secondary essays have been turned in (mid-late July) and before most interviews start (mid-late September). Of course, this timeline may shift depending on if you are applying to Texas schools, osteopathic (DO) programs, or early admission. Whatever your timeline, I suggest at least eight weeks of preparation. Thus, the book has been divided into eight sections, meant to be read and reviewed over an eight-week period.

Don't worry if you are reading this book less than eight weeks before your first interview. The content can still be useful on a shorter timeline and read in as little as a week. Powering through the book will mean a more intense experience and less time to research and practice, but you will nevertheless be able to improve your interview skills by reviewing the included questions, strategy, and insider tips.

This book contains a huge amount of information, gathered from my nearly 15 years of experience as a pre-med tutor and admissions consultant. But don't be intimidated! Using this book to guide your preparation will undoubtedly increase your chances of becoming an exceptional medical school interviewee.

Of course, this book will help you only as much as you are willing to practice. There is no way to memorize how to become a great interviewee. My goal for this book is to teach you strategies of how to prepare the best answers you are capable of delivering, instead of teaching you the exact wording of answers. Believe me, interviewers can see right through pre-meds who give over-rehearsed answers that don't feel genuine. I want you to be your best self on interview day. Using my strategies will provide the scaffolding on which to build your own interview voice. The ideal mix of interview preparation involves reading this book, doing the research suggested, performing mock interviews, practicing as much as possible, and staying true to yourself.

Though the book is geared to pre-meds applying through the AMCAS and TMDSAS systems, the allopathic and Texas applications respectively, the themes presented are also relevant to pre-meds applying to osteopathic (DO) and offshore schools. I have also included appendices discussing the unique aspects of DO and Caribbean admissions interviews.

Please note this book focuses on the "traditional" medical school interview. The Multiple Mini Interview (MMI) and the related online CASPer tests are certainly gaining momentum and rely heavily on ethical, group, and essay-writing scenarios. It follows that the sections of this book focusing on ethical and behavioral questions, as well as the discussions of group and essay questions, will be helpful for MMI preparation. But, as MMIs cover a broad range of topics and require a different approach to preparation when compared to "traditional" interviews, they are covered in another forthcoming e-book. Check back at www.MDadmit.com or www.howtobepremed.com for more information.

Acronyms

The medical school admissions process and this book are full of acronyms. I've placed them here for easy reference.

AMCAS	American Medical College Application Service
TMDSAS	Texas Medical & Dental Schools Application Service
OMSAS	Ontario Medical Schools Application Service
AACOMAS	American Association of Colleges of Osteopathic Medicine Application Service
AAMC	Association of American Medical Colleges
AACOM	American Association of Colleges of Osteopathic Medicine
MCAT	Medical College Admission Test
MD	Doctor of Medicine
DO	Doctor of Osteopathy
PhD	Doctor of Philosophy

Legal Disclaimer

I certainly cannot guarantee you success as a pre-med or admission to medical school by reading this book and following its advice. But I can assure your pre-med path will be less stressful and chances of medical school admission success will improve by learning interview preparation techniques.

Pardon the requisite legal verbiage:

The author/publisher of this book has used her best efforts in preparing this book. The author/publisher makes no representation or warranties with respect to the accuracy, applicability, fitness, or completeness of the contents of this book. The information contained in this book is strictly for educational purposes. Therefore, if you wish to apply ideas contained in this book, you are taking full responsibility for your actions. The author/publisher shall in no event be held liable to any party for any direct, indirect, punitive, special, incidental, or other consequential damages arising directly or indirectly from any use of this material, which is provided "as is" and without warranties.

The author/publisher does not warrant the performance, effectiveness, or applicability of any websites listed in this book. All websites are listed for information purposes only and are not warranted for content, accuracy, or any other implied or explicit purpose.

The author/publisher of this book made every effort to be as accurate and complete as possible in the creation of the book's content. However, due to the rapidly changing nature of medical school admissions, she does not warrant or represent at any time that the contents within are accurate. Application fees, dates, deadlines, websites, and addresses, in addition to admissions requirements, change every year, and it is the reader's responsibility to stay up-to-date on such changes.

The author/publisher will not be responsible for any losses or damages of any kind incurred by the reader whether directly or indirectly arising from the use of the information found in this book.

WEEK 1

The goal of this week is to ease you into medical school interview preparation by providing background on statistics, scheduling, interview types, and general interview preparation. Try not to be overwhelmed by the number of questions listed in Chapter 5. After reading this book, you will possess the strategy required to create outstanding answers to all of them.

Day 1
Read Chapters 1-3 (Statistics, Scheduling, and Interview Types)

Day 2
Read Chapter 4 (General Interview Preparation)

Day 3
Read Chapter 5 (Interview Questions Overview)
Skim the table of questions
Take a deep breath

Day 4
Read the first question from each of the 21 categories in Chapter 5 and answer each out loud off the top of your head

Day 5
Pick another question from each of the 21 categories in Chapter 5 and answer each out loud off the top of your head

Days 6-7
Put the book down and relax

CHAPTER 1

Statistics

I know. You think statistics are mundane and want to get right to practicing interview questions. But, as you will soon see, statistics provided by the AAMC can be very helpful when preparing for medical school interviews. Here's how the AAMC data derived from the survey mentioned in the preface can help us answer three very important questions regarding interviews.

1. How do medical schools decide who receives an interview?

Many pre-meds assume the majority of medical school admissions committees decide whom to interview based on a computer algorithm. Thankfully, this is a myth. According to the AAMC survey, which received responses from 90% of all admissions committees, only 12% used a computer algorithm to help select interview candidates. All other schools had admissions committee members or staff read the application. Yes, someone does actually review your AMCAS application and secondary essays (or TMDSAS for those Texas folks out there or AACOMAS for DO applicants). All that hard work writing your personal statement, choosing most meaningful activities, and answering diversity questions was not for naught!

2. *What characteristics are medical school admissions committees looking for during an interview?*

Thanks to this wonderful AAMC survey, we know exactly what qualities medical school admissions committees are evaluating during the interview. These are listed in order of frequency of response:

- Motivation for a medical career
- Compassion and empathy
- Personal maturity
- Oral communication
- Service orientation
- Professionalism
- Altruism
- Integrity
- Leadership
- Intellectual curiosity
- Teamwork
- Cultural competence
- Reliability and dependability
- Self-discipline
- Critical thinking
- Adaptability
- Verbal reasoning
- Work habits
- Persistence
- Resilience
- Logical reasoning

Isn't it fascinating how far down critical thinking and logical reasoning appear on this list? Admissions committees are not using interviews to test your knowledge of the Krebs Cycle or Newton's theories. That's what pre-med courses and the MCAT are supposed to do. Admissions committees want to evaluate your "soft" skills that cannot be learned in academic courses or assessed through standardized testing. It makes sense when you think about it. If medical schools just wanted to fill their limited seats with nerdy automatons who can recite the periodic table backwards, there would be no need for an interview. Look at law schools. They don't interview candidates and instead base admissions solely on grades, LSAT scores, recommendations, and a brief application. But medicine is different. It's a people profession at its core. And this is why the interview is so important. The admissions interviewer is trying to assess your capacity to be a compassionate, dedicated, and forward-thinking professional who works well with others, communicates effectively, and truly wants to dedicate your life to serving others. So even if you have a 4.0 GPA and 99th percentile MCAT, you still have to prepare just as hard for the interview as other pre-meds, and perhaps even harder. Medicine isn't just about brains. You need the whole package. The interview tests whether you are the real deal.

3. *What is the typical medical school interview process?*

It seems a lot is changing in medical school admissions these days. The MCAT2015 has arrived, many medical schools are turning to a "holistic" approach in admissions, and the Multiple Mini Interview (MMI) is rapidly gaining favor. A few years ago, a medical school interview probably involved one or two, thirty-minute sessions with either a professor or a professor and student. Now, interview processes range from "traditional" one-on-one interviews to group interviews to MMIs. And even if a school sticks with the traditional interview format, according to the AAMC survey, it is more likely to have a structured component, such as questions being provided to interviewers by the admissions committees. Unfortunately, schools shift their processes often, so new research is required each year to know what schools perform which kind of interview. Upon offering an interview invite, most medical schools inform the applicant of the interview type. This book will focus on the traditional medical school interview, which is still the most common type, and will also discuss ethical/behavioral questions, how to approach the group interview, and strategies for interview essay writing, tactics that will give you a head start on MMI preparation.

CHAPTER 2

Scheduling

Before we jump into details about the different types of interviews within the "traditional" category, I'd like to discuss scheduling. I am always amazed by how much angst interview scheduling causes pre-meds. Whole threads on Student Doctor Network (SDN) and other equally fretful Internet forums are devoted to determining the best time to interview and trying to game the system. Here's an insider secret. There is no hidden, complicated medical school interview scheduling system to game. The best time to interview is when you will be most prepared. Schedule your interviews when you will be fresh and ready to perform at the peak of your ability.

Most medical schools run interviews from September through March. Texas and DO schools often start as early as August. Receiving an early interview is a good sign, but doesn't guarantee admission. Similarly, an interview invite sent in January is just as important as one sent in September. If you haven't been offered an interview by January, it is unlikely, but not impossible, one will come your way (sorry for that harsh reality).

Scheduling has little bearing on interview acceptance chances except in rolling admissions schools. Rolling admissions schools interview a batch of applicants, and then offer the best candidates admission within weeks. The later you interview, the fewer spots will be available, and, generally speaking, the less likely you are to gain acceptance. Rolling admissions schools often take the scheduling decision out of your hands by providing one short window of interview dates. You simply need to choose the date that works best for you in the timeframe given. If you are offered a choice of interview dates many weeks to months apart, try to interview earlier rather than later. Of course, if you aren't going to be ready to interview during an earlier time frame, it's best to delay. A poor interview performance usually leads to rejection. It follows naturally that interviewing early and performing badly is worse than interviewing later and excelling, even at rolling admissions schools.

Remember, trying to interview early has no importance for regular admissions schools. There is no difference in your chance of acceptance if you interview in September or January. This is because most regular admission schools interview all candidates first, and then make final acceptance, waitlist, and rejection decisions sometime in February, March, or April. Take home point – scheduling should be based on what works best for you and your ability to shine.

A few other tidbits to consider when scheduling medical school interviews:

- Avoid interviewing at one of your top choice schools first if possible
- Don't schedule one of your top choice schools last in a long line of interviews when you could be burned out
- Plan sufficient time off for interview travel
- Arrive the night before the interview, so, if you are held up due to transportation problems, you will have adequate time to make secondary plans

CHAPTER 3

Interview Types

With the medical school interview landscape changing yearly, it is important to understand the different types of interviews you may be offered. The vast majority of medical schools will provide you with a brief overview of their general interview type along with the interview invitation. This critical information will allow you to best prepare for the interview day.

There are three main types of interviews:

1. Traditional interviews
2. Groups interviews
3. Multiple mini interviews (MMI)

TRADITIONAL INTERVIEWS

"Traditional" refers to the type of interviews most medical schools have been performing for years. These interviews are composed of one-on-one meetings with an admissions committee member for between 20 to 45 minutes. Most schools schedule two, one-on-one interviews on the interview day, usually involving two different professors or a professor and a student. Some schools provide only one interview, either with a professor or student, while others require up to five interviews. You don't have control over who interviews you and you are rarely provided interviewer names beforehand. Since it is inappropriate to request a specific interviewer, you will have to do the best with whomever you get.

The content of traditional interviews has changed over the years, but tends to be consistent as of late. Rarely are medical students grilled on their scientific knowledge or asked trick questions, as they were in the "old" days. When I applied, a story circulated about an interviewer who would leave the room and then have the phone ring. Whether you picked up the phone or not was part of the interview. These days, most medical schools ask their interviewers to gain a sense of the applicant's soft skills in attempt to predict a future physician's bedside manner and ability to work well with others. Thus, the tone of medical school interviews has relaxed tremendously. Sure, you may get a stick-in-the-mud of an interviewer who remembers being grilled when he applied to medical school and wants to pass this pain along to the future generation. But, in the vast majority of cases, interviewers try to foster comfortable and engaging conversations. Most medical applicants will tell you that 90% of their medical school interviews had a relaxed tone with straightforward questions.

MD/PhD candidates (along with other combined degree candidates) please note you will have multiple interviews, including separate sessions for each degree being pursued. The PhD interviews tend to be more formal and focused (and much less touchy-feely) than the MD interviews. PhD interviews are usually performed by MD/PhDs in the research field of your stated interest and are notorious for digging into deep detail about past and future research, from hypothesis formation to rigorous statistical methods and modeling. It is essential to know every aspect of the research listed on your application, even if you did not participate in each component of the investigation. Expect the MD/PhD interview day to include at least five interviews.

Most traditional interviews are "open," meaning the interviewer has read your full application (though how thoroughly the application has been read differs greatly from interviewer to interviewer). However, "closed" interviews, where the interviewer has not seen your application, are becoming more common. Less common are "semi-open" interviews where the interviewer has read only part of the application, such as the personal statement. Most medical schools will give you a heads up on whether they use open, semi-open, or closed interviews before the interview day.

GROUP INTERVIEWS

Group interviews are the least common interview type. They are used both for efficiency and to see how you handle a more intimidating situation. Group interviews come in two varieties:

1. Panel interview – you meet with multiple interviewers at once.
2. Colleague interview – you are interviewed with other applicants at the same time either by an individual or a group of interviewers.

The typical content of panel group interviews is similar to traditional interviews. Colleague interviews often ask the group to solve a problem or work together on an issue.

In a panel interview, address your answer to all the interviewers and not only the person who asked the question. You can often tell a panel interview is going well when an open conversation is created and interviewers feed off your response, engage with their colleagues, and even debate a point. Though it can seem chaotic, creating a situation that feels like a lively dinner table conversation usually means you are doing well.

As for interviews where other applicants are involved, try your best not to be intimidated. No matter how the other applicants present themselves, maintain your decorum, never interrupt, and stay true to your own opinions. Such group interviews are usually looking less at what you actually say and more at how you interact with others in the group. Though there is no need to be the loudest, it is important to have your voice heard in this type of group interview. Be sure to say something, hopefully brilliant, during an interview with colleagues.

MULTIPLE MINI INTERVIEWS (MMI)

The MMI format first showed up in the early 2000s. In brief, the MMI attempts to measure an applicant's soft skills through multiple stations posing different scenarios and each lasting about eight to ten minutes. Anything goes in a MMI, from an actor in the room to essay writing to group activities. Fortunately, many of the topics in this book, particularly the ethics and policy questions, group questions, and essay writing, can help with MMI preparation. Because it is so distinct from traditional interviews, I am writing a separate e-book dedicated to MMI preparation. Check back at www.MDadmit.com or www.howtobepremed.com for more information.

Stop here for today, as I want to ease you into interview preparation. Then move onto Chapter 4 tomorrow.

CHAPTER 4

General Interview Preparation

Now that you understand basic interview statistics, scheduling tips, and the different medical school interview types, we can jump into general preparation themes relevant to all interviews followed by an in-depth look at how to approach individual questions.

Let's start with the basics:

1. Know the interview type offered

If a medical school does not tell you its interview type in the invitation letter/e-mail, then check the school's website. If the information is not listed, call the admissions office and ask. Have you AAMC ID number ready in case the person who answers the phone wants to look up your application. Since I know many pre-meds get nervous calling admissions offices, here is a script you can follow:

> "Hello, my name is [insert your name here], and I am very excited to learn your school has offered me an interview. I am wondering if you could tell me the interview type and whether the interviews are open or closed file?"

Most admissions office staff will happily give you the details or tell you where to find them.

2. Research school

Hopefully, you have already thoroughly researched each school where you have applied. If this is the case, brush up on your knowledge by reviewing your notes. If you haven't researched the school in depth, do so prior to the interview. Start with the school's website and focus on its mission, curriculum, student body, patient population, affiliated hospitals, and location. Once you have obtained this basic knowledge, start looking for specifics about the school that interest you the most, such as student-run clinics, research labs, and elective opportunities. This information will be critical in answering school-specific interview questions, as you will see in Chapter 21.

3. Review AMCAS/TMDSAS and secondary applications

Given you likely spent many hours preparing your AMCAS and secondary applications, it may seem odd to suggest you review both of these frequently. However, you'd be surprised how easy it is to forget a class you took freshman year or an exact detail you mentioned on one secondary but not on another. Here are strategies you can follow when reviewing application materials:

Study all transcripts

Every course listed on all transcripts is fair game for the interviewer. You may have taken some of these classes four years ago (or, for some of you, 10+ years ago). Take notes on the professor's name, class topic, and highlights/lowlights. During one of my medical school interviews, the interviewer opened a folder containing my

AMCAS application, circled a finger over the transcript section, and dropped it on a class, saying, "Tell me about First Nights." Though First Nights was one of my very first college courses, I had prepared for such a question and happily explained the class studied the first performance of four classical music pieces. Had I not reviewed my transcript, I fear I would have looked like a deer in headlights upon being asked such a question.

Review work/activity list

For each activity listed, practice out loud describing your role and the experience's importance in one sentence. Pay special attention to your most meaningful experiences on the AMCAS application and why you chose them.

Read personal statement

The personal statement is your story and arguably the most important part of the primary application. Make sure you have your story down. I suggest reading your personal statement, and then pretending you have a 30-second elevator ride with an admissions committee member to summarize it. What would you say?

Know nuance of secondary essays

To reiterate the importance of reviewing the specific information you presented to each school, I will relay another story. While interviewing at Duke, the interviewer asked me what I wanted to do with the "extra" year (Duke squeezed the first two years of medical school into one year, freeing up a year to do research or obtain a second degree). I gave what I thought was a great answer about obtaining a MPH. The confused look on the interviewer's face should have tipped me off.

Turns out, I wrote my essay on how I would use the free year to continue studying the history of medicine, my college major. A quick reread of my Duke secondary essays would have prevented the mistake.

4. Stay up-to-date on current events

Many medical school interviewers weave current events into their questions, as it's only natural to ask about hot topics in the news. Stay up-to-date on all current events, especially those related to health care. Here are some tips on how to keep current on important events without spending hours every day reading newspapers.

Make your favorite news source the Internet browser home page

Whether it's the *New York Times, CNN, Huffington Post,* or *Reddit,* creating a news-oriented homepage will allow you to browse for interesting articles every time you open the web browser. Even 15 minutes of news browsing per day will make a positive impact on your knowledge of current events.

Save articles to a "read later" application

How many times a day do you see an interesting article or have a friend send you a video that you don't have time to read or watch? Instead of letting these interesting items pass by or fester in your e-mail inbox, post them to a read later application, such as Pocket, Instapaper, or Readability (or the many others that seem to pop up monthly). Simply hit a button on your web browser, and these apps compile all of your saved items in a central location to be accessed at any time on any of your devices (phone, tablet, computer). Save articles, websites, videos, and photos (only Pocket allows videos and photos at this time) throughout the week, and then spend an hour on

Sunday morning reading through your saved content over a cup of coffee or tea.

Read The Economist politics and business in review sections every week

These two short pages take less than 10 minutes to read and provide pertinent and succinct current event reviews. Subscribing to *The Economist* is pricey, but you can read these two sections at most university or public libraries.

5.   Brainstorm your opinions on common ethical topics

Ethical questions are becoming common parts of traditional interviews and make up the core of virtually every MMI. Ethical questions usually don't have right or wrong answers. Your opinion on moral topics is less important than the thought process driving you to form this opinion. In this book, I will walk through in detail the most common and most difficult ethical questions asked in medical school interviews. But a general way to prepare is to read about these topics, such as abortion, physician-assisted suicide, and cloning, as they come up in the news. By studying how others present their opinions on controversial ethical topics, you will be better able to form and communicate your own views.

6.   Practice, practice, and practice some more

The adage "practice makes perfect" could not be truer regarding medical school interviews. Even if you are a stellar candidate and natural interviewee, practice is essential to maximize interview performance. The bulk of this book discusses how to approach hundreds of interview questions. Take this question list and practice your answers out loud, preferably in front of a computer camera or mirror. Recording your answers is by far the most effective tactic. Just as athletes watch game tape to improve, you should watch interview tape to hone your technique. Pay attention not only to content, but also to distracting habits such as ring twirling, hand wringing, or foot tapping. Practice limiting distracting movements. Also look out for common verbal tics many of us turn to in moments of stress, including "um," "like," "sort of," "kind of," and "ya know." It will be painful to watch yourself on film, but it get's easier with (guess what?) practice!

Some applicants like to write down answers to questions first. This strategy works only if you then practice answering out loud without looking at the written notes. You want to sound polished but not like you are reciting a memorized answer.

Ideally, you should arrange a mock interview with a member of your school's pre-med committee and/or an admissions consultant. This mock interview should be as close to real as possible. Wear your suit, use an office setting, and answer each question to the best of your ability.

Here is a summary of interview tips you can refer to as you practice the questions in this book. I suggest bookmarking this list for future reference, and we will review the concepts listed as we move through the book.

- Humans think best in groups of three or less. Remember this "rule of threes" tactic.
- Tie answers to short personal anecdotes to keep the interviewer engaged and help her remember you.
- Keep answers to about a minute or less. Certain responses will require more than a minute, particularly policy and ethical/behavioral queries. In this era of immediate gratification, we often have short attention spans, and paying attention for more than a minute is challenging. Don't bore your interviewer. She can always ask follow-up questions if intrigued by a certain point.

- Refocus negative questions into a positive as quickly as possible.
- Tell the interviewer where you are going with your answers. Phrases such as, "I'd like to tell you my three main reasons," and, "I performed two significant projects I'd like to discuss" help the interviewer pay attention and remember your points.
- Avoid verbal tics, such as "um," "like," "sort of," "kind of," and "ya know." Be comfortable with short, silent pauses. Don't fill the air with throwaway words while you think. And please, please, please keep "like" to an absolute minimum.
- Policy and ethical/behavioral questions often require background knowledge. Do your homework to avoid being stumped on interview day.
- Stay true to yourself and your beliefs. Never guess what the interviewer wants to hear.
- Feel free to role play with the interviewer if the question lends itself to this approach.
- Practice, practice, practice. Practice in front of your computer and record the video. Watch and time yourself and be critical. Practice with parents, friends, pre-med tutors, admissions consultants, *etc.* Wear your suit during practice sessions to ensure it is comfortable.
- Don't memorize your answers. If you take notes, write down one-word or one-sentence reminders to trigger your memory. You want to strike a tone of preparedness but your answers should not appear over-rehearsed or memorized.
- Your goal is for the interview to feel like an engaging conversation.

Now that we've covered general interview preparation strategies, take a break for today. Tomorrow, we will move on to preparation for the most common and difficult questions you are likely to receive in medical school interviews.

CHAPTER 5

Interview Questions Overview

Over the past 10+ years, I have gathered interview questions from many sources to help my clients prepare for the interview day. These sources include post-interview discussions with pre-meds, chats with fellow professors about questions they ask, social media discussions, and searching websites such as aamc.org and forums like Student Doctor Network and Old Premeds. Although new questions emerge every year, it became clear while creating my master interview question list that most queries fit into one of 21 general categories. Though there are infinite numbers of questions you can be asked during a medical school interview, there are only so many categories interviewers can choose from. This is a key point in medical school interview preparation. You don't have time to prepare for limitless possible questions, but you can certainly develop a strategy for answering 21 categories of questions.

I have listed below over 250 interview questions in random fashion. When you read through the list, I bet you will feel overwhelmed. I certainly did when I first read it. Move on to the next list, where I have grouped the same questions into 21 categories. Immediately, you will see how much easier it is for the brain to process these questions. This strategy of categorization will be essential to your interview preparation, as you will learn how one answer can be used to respond to many different questions with only minor tweaks.

For those of you who have read *The Medical School Admissions Guide*, the technique of adapting one answer for multiple purposes will sound familiar. This is exactly how I suggest secondary essays be tackled. Just as you should create 10-15 stellar essays to answer the most common and difficult secondary essay prompts, so you should devise a set of responses to answer questions in the most common and difficult medical school interview question categories. Instead of teaching you how to best answer every one of the 250+ questions listed below, I will show you how to think about each category of questions and strategize excellent responses that can be used over and over to impress your interviewers.

Interview Question List (Sorted Randomly)

Tell me about yourself.
Why do you want to be a doctor?
A three-year-old female arrives in your emergency department unresponsive and with unstable vital signs. There is no adult available to consent for life-saving treatment. What do you do?
Do you think your volunteer work makes a real difference?
Why did you choose your undergraduate institution?
How will you handle the stress of medical school?
The son of a patient is a physician and calls you to discuss his father's case. What do you say?
What are your strengths?
What are your weaknesses?
What was your childhood like?

Which clinical experience did you find most impactful?

What was something you learned for fun?

Give me three positives and three negatives about the Affordable Care Act.

Rate your humbleness on a scale of 1-10.

Define pain without examples to a six year old.

What values do you bring from your cultural background that will be useful in medicine?

Do you think healthcare should be rationed?

Define empathy and give an example.

What is the biggest mistake you have ever made, and what did you learn from it?

Assume your hospital has regulations about the number of hours you can work per day, and you have already worked the maximum number of hours allowed. What would you do if one of your patients coded at the end of your shift?

A small town has a sudden surge in DUI and alcohol-related arrests. How would you go about researching the root of the problem?

Where do you see yourself in 10 years?

Medicine is a depressing business - how will you cope?

Where else have you interviewed?

What would you like me to know?

Provide me with an example of your leadership ability.

You are on the organ transplant committee and have to choose between two individuals with liver damage who will die if they don't receive a new liver a) A 35-year-old mother with three children all below the age of 6 and a history of drug abuse b) A 50-year-old man with 20-year-old twins and a history of alcohol abuse. This person's family has given large donations to the school.

A fourth-year medical student close to graduation messes up (ethically). What would you do to discipline him?

If you had $100,000 that could support one cancer patient or 100 healthy patients, how would you allocate the funds?

Tell me a joke.

What class impressed you the most positively or negatively in your undergraduate education?

How have you served the community?

What do you hope to get out of medicine?

Tell me about your most meaningful extracurricular experience.

When did you first become interested in medicine?

What TV character is most like your personality?

If a doctor is the coach of a sport, what sport do you think best fits and why?

What would you do if you unknowingly resuscitated a DNR patient?

Tell me about the lowest point in your life.

Should we mandate HIV testing?

I see your father/mother is a doctor. Prove to me you are not going into medicine to please him/her/them.

Would you ever lie to a patient?

If you were the head of so and so company and we gave you 100 billion dollars, how would you allocate the money?

You are caring for a patient you believe has no chance of meaningful survival. The family requests you do everything you can to save her. You have already put the patient on full life support and want to stop with the resuscitation, as you believe the care is futile. What do you do?

Why did you obtain a graduate degree?

In 25 years, looking back on your medical career, how will you determine if you have been successful?

Tell me about an experience during your shadowing that made you uncomfortable.

There seems to be a mismatch between your GPA and MCAT. Please explain.

What does diversity mean to you?

What specialty are you considering?

What do you do to blow off steam?

Define professionalism.

Name some good qualities you possess and one quality you'd like to work on or change.

What is your passion?

Describe a time you needed to ask for help.

Why [insert school name]?

If you could have dinner with three people, living or dead, who would they be and why?

If you were a cereal (animal, book, tree, dessert, kitchen utensil, *etc.*), what kind of cereal would you be and why?

How should we deal with "bad" doctors?

What do you think about genetic testing for [insert disease name]? (assume non-curable, life-threatening disease)?

I understand there are no/few doctors in your family. How do you know it's the right profession for you?

Have you ever been discriminated against?

As a medical student, you are asked to consent an elderly woman for a hernia repair. She can barely hear and you are fairly confident she didn't understand the consent. When you tell the senior resident of your issue, she says, "Just get it done." What do you do?

When was the last time you felt humbled?

Have you ever harmed anyone?

What is your greatest academic achievement?

You are caring for an unconscious patient unable to provide consent regarding release of information to his family. His brother calls you to ask how the patient is doing. What do you say?

What was your most memorable physician shadowing experience?

Think about the people you don't like. What don't you like about them?

What is the role of physicians in society?

Has anyone attempted to dissuade you from becoming a physician? If so, how did you respond?

Tell me about your family/upbringing.

Tell me about the most interesting case you have seen.

Are you involved in the arts in any way?

Tell me something I can't find anywhere on your application.

Is medicine a service profession?

What is one question you wish we had asked you? Please answer it.

Have you ever been overwhelmed? How did you handle this?

Did you have an "aha" moment when you decided medicine was the career for you?

What would you like written in your obituary?

Why should we admit you?

Tell me about your research.

Why are you in a sorority/fraternity?

What was a time you made a poor choice?

Are you involved in sports?

Do you ever think about your own mortality?

Do mid-level providers who obtain PhD's have the right to call themselves "Doctor" in a clinical setting?

What was your favorite college course and why?

Describe a time when you thought it was better to be dishonest than to tell the truth.

What kind of medical problems will we face on Mars?

You three have just moved into a one-bedroom apartment together. Take 10 minutes to plan out how you are going to live with each other.

How do you feel about euthanasia?

How will you add to the diversity of this school?

What do you think are the biggest challenges facing the healthcare system today?

You are a fourth-year resident performing research and preparing to present your data at an upcoming global conference. Just before you leave, you discover your principal investigator (PI) is falsifying data. What do you do?

What was your least favorite college course and why?

What are your hobbies?

How do you feel advancements in gene therapy will affect the future of medicine?

Tell me a funny story.

Describe a time when you let someone down and how you resolved the situation.

You are an emergency physician caring for a cardiac arrest patient who was brought in by ambulance from a supermarket. As the patient arrives, you receive a call from his daughter stating she has a DNR order and is bringing it in immediately. At the same time, the patient's son arrives in the ED and demands you do everything possible to save his father. What do you do?

Do you feel your undergraduate education has challenged you?

Where do you see the state of healthcare going over the next 10 years?

How will you change the world?

Is there anything else you would like me to know?

How would you fix healthcare?

Tell me about your publications.

What would you do differently?

What was your most meaningful community service experience?

Who has been a mentor in your life?

What do you find frustrating?

If you were to change one thing about the future what would it be?

Describe the ideal physician.

Pretend you've been working and studying nonstop for weeks and you finally have a day off. What do you do with it?

Do you think the MCAT is a good measure or determining factor for admission to medical school?

Describe your undergraduate education.

Pretend you are at a conference presenting your most important research, and I am in the audience. Give me your presentation.

Tell me about a time when a physician acted inappropriately. How did you react?

What do you think about cloning?

Give me an example of a time when you were on a team and it didn't work out.

Why doctor and not PA, NP, or RN?

What are you most ashamed of?

How will you handle a patient refusing treatment you have recommended?

What do you think about a public option for health insurance?

What is the most impactful research you have done?

What makes you laugh?

Do you feel you have had to overcome any hardships/struggles?

Would you ever perform an abortion? If so, under what circumstances?

How will you deal with leaving your family and moving to a new location?

Why is your research not published?

If your attending came into work intoxicated but still performed his work well, would you report him?

What is your biggest regret in life?

At what point do you as a physician stop devoting time and resources to a terminally-ill patient?

A 15-year old girl with a two-year-old child presents with a broken arm and requires surgery. The 15-year-old's guardian is not available to consent for the surgery. What do you do?

Think about people who don't like you. What would they say about you?

If [insert school name] was theoretically your first choice school, what would be your second choice school?

Why did you choose your undergraduate major?

Do you think we should have universal healthcare?

If you could go back in time and ask Henrietta Lacks for permission to use her cells, would you?

If you were given a $1 million grant to perform research, what would you do with it?

Are you a crammer or do you study a little each day?

What do you think about the current state of malpractice in the US?

What labs or research institutions at this school particularly interest you?

Describe a time you were in a minority.

Would you treat an illegal alien?

Prove to me you know what it's like to be a doctor.

What do you think accounts for the high cost of healthcare?

What do you do for exercise?

How would your brother/sister/cousin describe you?

What challenges do you expect to encounter as a physician?

Tell me about your service trip abroad.

If you could not be a doctor, what would you do?

Tell me about your graduate studies.

What is the hardest question you have ever been asked? How did you answer it?

A pharmacist refused to give birth control to a patient with a valid prescription citing ethical beliefs. What do you think about this?

I work for TIME Magazine and am in charge of selecting the person of the year. Whom would you nominate and why?

What do you think about health insurance mandates?

In what environment do you learn best?

Would you rather be a compassionate or a competent physician?

A 16-year-old female, whom you have known and treated in addition to her family for 10+ years, comes to you asking for a birth control prescription. How do you handle this?

What drives you?

If you were president, what would your health reform bill look like?

Do you really think a two-week service trip made a real difference to the community you served?

If you could go back and improve one area of your application, what would it be and why?

If you were given a million dollars, what would you do with it?

Tell me about a time when you had to assert yourself.

Describe a time when you were a patient and received medical care. What did you learn from the experience?

If a patient were brain dead and on life support, how would you make the decision whether or not to discontinue life support?

Give an example of a time you changed your position on a topic. Why?

Would you operate on a HIV+ patient that requires a minor knee operation?

As a re-applicant, how have you improved your application?

You are a primary care physician who has cared for Mrs. Mitchell for 30 years. She has been diagnosed with terminal cancer and comes into your office asking for pills she can take when she is ready to die. How do you respond?

How do you manage your time?

My house is infested with chipmunks. What should I do?

What does being a leader mean to you?

What's the difference between talent and skill?

Medical mistakes are common but not always important. Significant errors leading to morbidity, such as leaving a sponge in the abdomen after surgery, must be disclosed to patients. Should physicians also disclose less important mistakes, such a single inconsequential medication error?

What is the worst thing that has ever happened to you?

Do you think money is better spent researching HIV/AIDS treatment or cancer treatment?

What's the best advice you have ever been given?

If you could change one thing about the Affordable Care Act (Obamacare), what would it be?

How would you deal with a patient who is non-compliant?

Describe a time in which you failed at something in a non-academic setting.

Of a seven-year-old girl with Down Syndrome, a 35-year-old single man with a former drug addiction, and a 51-year-old man with a wife and two children, to whom would you give a heart if you only had one?

What is the most interesting fact you know?

Create a reality show where the winner gets a full ride to medical school.

If you are not accepted into medical school this year, what will you do?

Who is your idol/inspiration and why?

Have you ever seen someone die? How did you handle this?

You are a first year med student. At a party one of your classmates has six beers in one hour and gets really drunk. He behaves similarly at the next party and ends up punching someone. How would you handle the situation?

Define success.

A 13-year-old boy presents with "leaking" from his penis, and you diagnose him with a STD. He begs you not to tell his parents. What do you do beyond prescribing him the correct medication?

How do you feel your religious beliefs will influence your patient care?

Do you have any biases?

If you walked into a room with a block of stone and a chisel and were asked to carve an idea or concept, what would you carve and why?

What are you looking for in a medical school?

Mrs. Chang is an 80-year-old Asian woman who was hit by a car and is seriously injured. You are the ICU doctor in charge. As you enter Mrs. Chang's room to tell her the diagnosis, her son stops you and requests you do not to tell her the diagnosis as it will be upsetting and prevent her from getting better. He will make all of the medical decisions. What do you do?

Explain your poor grades [insert semester/year here].

If the president approached you to help solve a local obesity problem, how would you go about making a difference in the community?

Describe a personal conflict you've had with somebody and how you dealt with it.

What test(s) would you give to a teenage girl who wants an abortion?

Name five words off the top of your head that describe you.

You are taking care of a child who is seriously injured after a car accident with an actively bleeding spleen requiring a blood transfusion. The parents refuse to consent for the child to receive a blood transfusion given their religious beliefs. What do you do?

How would you teach someone who doesn't speak English to use a toothbrush?

What if while you are spending more time with a terminally-ill elderly patient, you spend less time with a sick child, miss a diagnosis, and the child dies?

How did your study abroad experience affect you and your studies?

Many IRBs stipulate that researchers in developing countries provide the same standard of care for patients as they do in the US. What do you think about this stipulation?

A patient who has signed a DNR order has changed her mind and verbally requests you do everything possible to keep her alive. What do you do?

A woman with chronic pain and known narcotic addiction presents in your office requesting medications. She refuses to leave until you give her narcotics. What do you do?

Define maturity.

Would you have "pulled the plug" on Terri Schiavo?

At [insert school name here], we work with underserved populations such as Hispanics and African Americans. Have you had experience with underserved populations?

How would you handle being unable to help someone or making a serious clinical mistake?

How do you reconcile your religious faith and interest in science?

If the military draft was reactivated and you were drafted tomorrow into the army, what would you do?

Mr. Anderson is dying and in a lot of pain. You want to give him morphine, but the medication will likely lower his blood pressure and hasten his death. You've exhausted all your options. Mr. Anderson is still in pain and wants you to end his life. What do you do?

What are you most proud of that is not on your resume?

What do you think the term Obamacare means?

If your classmate had to miss a class and asked you to sign him in for credit, what would you say to him?

How do you know you will enjoy taking care of sick people?

How do you think we can decrease medical errors?

The state you are practicing in passes a law requiring you to ask the citizenship status of all of your patients, and then turn this information into the state at the end of every month. What do you do?

Do you expect to continue performing research during medical school?

If you could go back and relive one day in your life, what day would that be? Would you change something about it? If so, what?

Describe your ideal medical school.

Explain to a six year old how to tie shoes without using hand gestures.

I am the governor, and my wife wants to spend millions on an anti-meth campaign. What do you think about this use of funds?

Name a time when you saw someone acting unprofessionally. What did you do and why?

What do you think will be the next great global medical breakthrough?

Tell me about the institutional action against you. How have you changed since then?

Name one situation that impacted you the most.

Imagine you are on trial and we are the jury. Try to convince us you are compassionate and empathetic.

If you got into Harvard or UCSF, would you come here?

How can we work to reduce the discrepancies in health care delivery in different areas of the city/state/country?

Describe a time you misjudged someone.

You walk into the room of a Haitian patient who has had a stroke and is not to eat or drink. The room is filled with his family members who are feeding him and none of them speak English. What do you do?

What do you do for fun?

What has been your most defining moment?

If your sister's boyfriend came to your practice with a STD, what would you do?

What research have you done and why?

What is your favorite book (movie, magazine *etc.*) and why?

What technology do you believe will have the biggest impact on healthcare in the next 10 years?

Name five things you can do with a pencil other than use it to write or draw.

What other schools have you applied to?

Can you tell me about a book that changed your perspective on life?

If a thoracic surgeon visited his patients prior to surgery and read from his bible to try and "save" them in case any troubles arose, how would you respond?

What happened on the MCAT?

What do you love?

What do/did you spend most of your time doing outside the classroom?

A 13-year-old girl is diagnosed with Hodgkin's. Her parents refuse what you believe is life-saving treatment for her and decide to travel out of the country for alternative, experimental therapies. What do you do?

What do you want me to say about you to the admissions board?

How would your friends describe you?

What do you think about pharmaceutical direct advertising to physicians? To patients? (TV ads, radio ads, mailings, *etc.*)

I'm visiting your state/school, and I've never been there before. Where would you take me?

In an operating room, there's the surgeon, anesthesiologist, nurses, technicians, *etc.* Who is the most important person in that room?

Should it be legal to force someone, who has shown signs of harming himself or herself or someone else, to take medication?

You are seeing a patient with kidney failure who refuses dialysis. He later loses consciousness, and his family requests that you dialyze immediately. What do you say and do?

How would you recommend alleviating the shortage of primary care doctors in certain areas of the US?

How do you work with a teammate who is not pulling his or her weight?

You are caring for a pregnant woman on life support. The child's life is in jeopardy and delivery is urgently needed, but the husband won't agree to the procedure. What do you do?

When were you glad you gave someone a second chance?

What makes you angry?

Why not go to your state school where tuition is cheaper?

Tell me about a time you felt misjudged by somebody, and how you responded to that situation.

If you were accepted to all the schools where you applied, how would you decide which school to attend?

Is it acceptable for physicians to modify medical information on insurance forms so companies will be more likely to reimburse patients?

A seven-year-old boy has presented to your emergency department for the sixth time this month, and you find out his mother has been neglecting to give him his meds. What do you do?

What is your top choice medical school?

Describe a specific time you helped someone in the last two weeks.

What do you think are the three most pressing public health issues facing the US today?

What are your thoughts on alternative medicine?

Your patient requires gallbladder surgery and speaks only Thai. You do not speak Thai, and there are no interpreters available in the hospital. What do you do?

Do you think the US should have a national medical errors database? Why or why not?

If you were crashed on a desert island with a group of natives who worship wooden idols, and the pilot has a broken leg that is bleeding, what 5 items that are common to luggage would you want to have and why?

Interview Questions List (Category)

I. Motivation for Medicine

1. Why do you want to be a doctor?

2. When did you first become interested in medicine?

3. Did you have an "aha" moment when you decided medicine was the career for you?

4. Why doctor and not PA, NP, or RN?

5. I see your father/mother is a doctor. Prove to me you are not going into medicine to please him/her/them.

6. I understand there are no/few doctors in your family. How do you know it's the right profession for you?

7. What do you hope to get out of medicine?

8. Has anyone attempted to dissuade you from becoming a physician? If so, how did you respond?

9. If you could not be a doctor, what would you do?

II. Open-ended

10. Tell me about yourself.

11. What was your childhood like?

12. Tell me about your family/upbringing.

13. What would you like me to know?

14. Tell me something I can't find anywhere on your application.

15. What is one question you wish we had asked you? Please answer it.

16. Is there anything else you would like me to know?

III. Academics

17. Why did you choose your undergraduate institution?

18. Why did you choose your undergraduate major?

19. What was your favorite college course and why?

20. What was your least favorite college course and why?

21. What class impressed you the most positively or negatively in your undergraduate education?

22. Do you feel your undergraduate education has challenged you?

23. Describe your undergraduate education.

24. What is your greatest academic achievement?

25. Are you a crammer or do you study a little each day?

26. In what environment do you learn best?

27. What was something you learned for fun?

28. How did your study abroad experience affect you and your studies?

29. Why did you obtain a graduate degree?

30. Tell me about your graduate studies.

IV. Research

31. Tell me about your research.

32. What research have you done and why?

33. What is the most impactful research you have done?

34. Pretend you are at a conference presenting your most important research, and I am in the audience. Give me your presentation.

35. Do you expect to continue performing research during medical school?

36. What labs or research institutions at this school particularly interest you?

37. Tell me about your publications.

38. Why is your research not published?

39. If you were given a $1 million grant to perform research, what would you do with it?

V. Service

40. How have you served the community?

41. What was your most meaningful community service experience?

42. Do you think your volunteer work makes a real difference?

43. Describe a specific time you helped someone in the last two weeks.

44. Tell me about your service trip abroad.

45. Do you really think a two-week service trip made a real difference to the community you served?

46. Is medicine a service profession?

VI. Extracurricular/Well-rounded

47. What do/did you spend most of your time doing outside the classroom?

48. Tell me about your most meaningful extracurricular experience.

49. What do you do for fun?

50. What are your hobbies?

51. Pretend you've been working and studying nonstop for weeks and you finally have a day off. What do you do with it?

52. Why are you in a sorority/fraternity?

53. Are you involved in the arts in any way?

54. Are you involved in sports?

55. What do you do for exercise?

VII. Clinical Experience

56. Which clinical experience did you find most impactful?

57. What was your most memorable physician shadowing experience?

58. Tell me about the most interesting case you have seen.

59. Prove to me you know what it's like to be a doctor.

60. Tell me about an experience during your shadowing that made you uncomfortable.

61. Describe a time when you were a patient and received medical care. What did you learn from the experience?

VIII. Application-related

62. Explain your poor grades [insert semester/year here].

63. What happened on the MCAT?

64. There seems to be a mismatch between your GPA and MCAT. Please explain.

65. Do you think the MCAT is a good measure or determining factor for admission to medical school?

66. Tell me about the institutional action against you. How have you changed since then?

67. If you could go back and improve one area of your application, what would it be and why?

68. As a re-applicant, how have you improved your application?

69. If you are not accepted into medical school this year, what will you do?

70. What other schools have you applied to?

71. Where else have you interviewed?

IX. Future

72. Where do you see yourself in 10 years?

73. What specialty are you considering?

74. In 25 years, looking back on your medical career, how will you determine if you have been successful?

75. If you were to change one thing about the future what would it be?

X. Diversity

76. What does diversity mean to you?

77. How will you add to the diversity of this school?

78. Describe a time you were in a minority.

79. What values do you bring from your cultural background that will be useful in medicine?

80. At [insert school name here], we work with underserved populations such as Hispanics and African Americans. Have you had experience with underserved populations?

XI. Coping Skills

81. Medicine is a depressing business - how will you cope?

82. How will you handle the stress of medical school?

83.	What do you do to blow off steam?
84.	How do you know you will enjoy taking care of sick people?
85.	Have you ever seen someone die? How did you handle this?
86.	How would you handle being unable to help someone or making a serious clinical mistake?
87.	How will you deal with leaving your family and moving to a new location?
88.	Have you ever been overwhelmed? How did you handle this?

XII. Professionalism/Physician Role

89.	Define professionalism.
90.	Describe the ideal physician.
91.	What is the role of physicians in society?
92.	Tell me about a time when a physician acted inappropriately. How did you react?
93.	Name a time when you saw someone acting unprofessionally. What did you do and why?
94.	In an operating room, there's the surgeon, anesthesiologist, nurses, technicians, *etc.* Who is the most important person in that room?
95.	If a doctor is the coach of a sport, what sport do you think best fits and why?

XIII. Characteristics

96.	What are your strengths?
97.	What are your weaknesses?
98.	Name some good qualities you possess and one quality you'd like to work on or change.
99.	Name five words off the top of your head that describe you.

100.	How would your friends describe you?
101.	How would your brother/sister/cousin describe you?
102.	Think about people who don't like you. What would they say about you?
103.	Think about the people you don't like. What don't you like about them?

XIV. Soft Skills/Inner Self

104.	Provide me with an example of your leadership ability.
105.	What does being a leader mean to you?
106.	How do you manage your time?
107.	Rate your humbleness on a scale of 1-10.
108.	What's the difference between talent and skill?
109.	Define success.
110.	Define empathy and give an example.
111.	Define maturity.
112.	What are you most proud of that is not on your resume?
113.	What has been your most defining moment?
114.	Name one situation that impacted you the most.
115.	What is your passion?
116.	What do you love?
117.	What drives you?
118.	What makes you laugh?
119.	What makes you angry?
120.	What do you find frustrating?
121.	Do you have any biases?
122.	Would you rather be a compassionate or a competent physician?

XV. Challenge

123.	What is the biggest mistake you have ever made, and what did you learn from it?
124.	Do you feel you have had to overcome any hardships/struggles?
125.	What are you most ashamed of?
126.	What is your biggest regret in life?
127.	Describe a time in which you failed at something in a non-academic setting.
128.	What was a time you made a poor choice?
129.	Describe a time when you let someone down and how you resolved the situation.
130.	Describe a personal conflict you've had with somebody and how you dealt with it.
131.	If you could go back and relive one day in your life, what day would that be? Would you change something about it? If so, what?
132.	Tell me about the lowest point in your life.
133.	What is the worst thing that has ever happened to you?
134.	How do you work with a teammate who is not pulling his or her weight?
135.	Give me an example of a time when you were on a team and it didn't work out? What would you do differently?
136.	When were you glad you gave someone a second chance?
137.	Tell me about a time you felt misjudged by somebody, and how you responded to that situation.
138.	Describe a time you misjudged someone.
139.	Have you ever been discriminated against?
140.	When was the last time you felt humbled?

141.	Have you ever harmed anyone?
142.	Describe a time you needed to ask for help.
143.	Tell me about a time when you had to assert yourself.
144.	What challenges do you expect to encounter as a physician?
145.	What is the hardest question you have ever been asked? How did you answer it?

XVI. School Specific

146.	Why [insert school name]?
147.	What are you looking for in a medical school?
148.	Describe your ideal medical school.
149.	Why not go to your state school where tuition is cheaper?
150.	If you were accepted to all the schools where you applied, how would you decide which school to attend?
151.	If you got into Harvard or UCSF, would you come here?
152.	What is your top choice medical school?
153.	If [insert school name] was theoretically your first choice school, what would be your second choice school?

XVII. Sell Yourself

154.	What do you want me to say about you to the admissions board?
155.	Why should we admit you?
156.	What would you like written in your obituary?
157.	How will you change the world?
158.	Imagine you are on trial and we are the jury. Try to convince us you are compassionate and empathetic.

XVIII. Outside the Box

159.	If you were a cereal (animal, book, tree, dessert, kitchen utensil, *etc.*), what kind of cereal would you be and why?
160.	What TV character is most like your personality?
161.	If you walked into a room with a block of stone and a chisel and were asked to carve an idea or concept, what would you carve and why?
162.	If you were given a million dollars, what would you do with it?
163.	If the military draft was reactivated and you were drafted tomorrow into the army, what would you do?
164.	What is your favorite book (movie, magazine *etc.*) and why?
165.	Can you tell me about a book that changed your perspective on life?
166.	Who is your idol/inspiration and why?
167.	I work for *TIME Magazine* and am in charge of selecting the person of the year. Whom would you nominate and why?
168.	If you could have dinner with three people, living or dead, who would they be and why?
169.	Who has been a mentor in your life?
170.	Tell me a joke.
171.	Tell me a funny story.
172.	What's the best advice you have ever been given?
173.	What is the most interesting fact you know?
174.	Give an example of a time you changed your position on a topic. Why?
175.	Explain to a six year old how to tie shoes without using hand gestures.
176.	Define pain without examples to a six year old.

177.	How would you teach someone who doesn't speak English to use a toothbrush?
178.	I'm visiting your state/school, and I've never been there before. Where would you take me?
179.	Name five things you can do with a pencil other than use it to write or draw.
180.	My house is infested with chipmunks. What should I do?
181.	Do you ever think about your own mortality?
182.	Do mid-level providers who obtain PhD's have the right to call themselves "Doctor" in a clinical setting?
183.	What kind of medical problems will we face on Mars?

XIX. Policy/Health System/Public Health

184.	What do you think are the biggest challenges facing the healthcare system today?
185.	Where do you see the state of healthcare going over the next 10 years?
186.	How would you fix healthcare?
187.	If you could change one thing about the Affordable Care Act (Obamacare), what would it be?
188.	Give me three positives and three negatives about the Affordable Care Act.
189.	What do you think the term Obamacare means?
190.	What do you think about a public option for health insurance?
191.	What do you think about health insurance mandates?
192.	Do you think we should have universal healthcare?
193.	If you were president, what would your health reform bill look like?

194.	What do you think accounts for the high cost of healthcare?
195.	If the president approached you to help solve a local obesity problem, how would you go about making a difference in the community?
196.	How would you recommend alleviating the shortage of primary care doctors in certain areas of the US?
197.	What do you think are the three most pressing public health issues facing the US today?
198.	How can we work to reduce the discrepancies in health care delivery in different areas of the city/state/country?
199.	What are your thoughts on alternative medicine?
200.	What technology do you believe will have the biggest impact on healthcare in the next 10 years?
201.	What do you think will be the next great global medical breakthrough?

XX. Ethical/Behavioral

A. Maternal/Fetal Conflict

202.	Would you ever perform an abortion? If so, under what circumstances?
203.	What test(s) would you give to a teenage girl who wants an abortion?
204.	You are caring for a pregnant woman on life support. The child's life is in jeopardy and delivery is urgently needed, but the husband won't agree to the procedure. What do you do?

B. End-of-Life Care/Physician Aid-in-Dying/Euthanasia

205.	How do you feel about euthanasia?

206. You are a primary care physician who has cared for Mrs. Mitchell for 30 years. She has been diagnosed with terminal cancer and comes into your office asking for pills she can take when she is ready to die. How do you respond?

207. Mr. Anderson is dying and in a lot of pain. You want to give him morphine, but the medication will likely lower his blood pressure and hasten his death. You've exhausted all your options. Mr. Anderson is still in pain and wants you to end his life. What do you do?

208. At what point do you as a physician stop devoting time and resources to a terminally-ill patient?

C. Do Not Resuscitate (DNR) Orders

209. What would you do if you unknowingly resuscitated a DNR patient?

210. You are an emergency physician caring for a cardiac arrest patient who was brought in by ambulance from a supermarket. As the patient arrives, you receive a call from his daughter stating she has a DNR order and is bringing it in immediately. At the same time, the patient's son arrives in the ED and demands you do everything possible to save his father. What do you do?

211. A patient who has signed a DNR order has changed her mind and verbally requests you do everything possible to keep her alive. What do you do?

D. Termination of Life-Sustaining Treatment/Futility

212. If a patient were brain dead and on life support, how would you make the decision whether or not to discontinue life support?

213. Would you have "pulled the plug" on Terri Schiavo?

214. You are caring for a patient you believe has no chance of meaningful survival. The family requests you do everything you can to save her. You have already put the patient on full life support and want to stop with the resuscitation, as you believe the care is futile. What do you do?

E. Spirituality in Medicine/Cross-Cultural Issues

215. How do you reconcile your religious faith and interest in science?

216. How do you feel your religious beliefs will influence your patient care?

217. You are taking care of a child who is seriously injured after a car accident with an actively bleeding spleen requiring a blood transfusion. The parents refuse to consent for the child to receive a blood transfusion given their religious beliefs. What do you do?

218. A pharmacist refused to give birth control to a patient with a valid prescription citing ethical beliefs. What do you think about this?

219. If a thoracic surgeon visited his patients prior to surgery and read from his bible to try and "save" them in case any troubles arose, how would you respond?

220. You walk into the room of a Haitian patient who has had a stroke and is not to eat or drink. The room is filled with his family members who are feeding him and none of them speak English. What do you do?

F. Truth-Telling and Withholding Information

221. Would you ever lie to a patient?

222. Describe a time when you thought it was better to be dishonest than to tell the truth.

223. Mrs. Chang is an 80-year-old Asian woman who was hit by a car and is seriously injured. You are the ICU doctor in charge. As you enter Mrs. Chang's room to tell her the diagnosis, her son stops you and requests you do not to tell her the diagnosis as it will be upsetting and prevent her from getting better. He will make all of the medical decisions. What do you do?

224. Is it acceptable for physicians to modify medical information on insurance forms so companies will be more likely to reimburse patients?

G. Professionalism

225. How should we deal with "bad" doctors?

226. If your attending came into work intoxicated but still performed his work well, would you report him?

227. You are a first year med student. At a party one of your classmates has six beers in one hour and gets really drunk. He behaves similarly at the next party and ends up punching someone. How would you handle the situation?

228. If your classmate had to miss a class and asked you to sign him in for credit, what would you say to him?

229. Assume your hospital has regulations about the number of hours you can work per day, and you have already worked the maximum number of hours allowed. What would you do if one of your patients coded at the end of your shift?

H. Doctor-Patient Relationship

230. How would you deal with a patient who is non-compliant?

231. The state you are practicing in passes a law requiring you to ask the citizenship status of all of your patients, and then turn this information into the state at the end of every month. What do you do?

232.	Would you treat an illegal alien?
233.	What do you think about pharmaceutical direct advertising to physicians? To patients? (TV ads, radio ads, mailings, *etc.*)
234.	A woman with chronic pain and known narcotic addiction presents in your office requesting medications. She refuses to leave until you give her narcotics. What do you do?

I. Refusal of Care/Parental Decision Making

235.	How will you handle a patient refusing treatment you have recommended?
236.	A 13-year-old girl is diagnosed with Hodgkin's. Her parents refuse what you believe is life-saving treatment for her and decide to travel out of the country for alternative, experimental therapies. What do you do?
237.	A seven-year-old boy has presented to your emergency department for the sixth time this month, and you find out his mother has been neglecting to give him his meds. What do you do?
238.	Should it be legal to force someone, who has shown signs of harming himself or herself or someone else, to take medication?
239.	You are seeing a patient with kidney failure who refuses dialysis. He later loses consciousness, and his family requests that you dialyze immediately. What do you say and do?

J. Confidentiality

| 240. | If your sister's boyfriend came to your practice with a STD, what would you do? |
| 241. | The son of a patient is a physician and calls you to discuss his father's case. What do you say? |

242. You are caring for an unconscious patient unable to provide consent regarding release of information to his family. His brother calls you to ask how the patient is doing. What do you say?

K. Care of Minors/Emancipated Minors

243. A 16-year-old female, whom you have known and treated in addition to her family for 10+ years, comes to you asking for a birth control prescription. How do you handle this?

244. A 13-year-old boy presents with "leaking" from his penis, and you diagnose him with a STD. He begs you not to tell his parents. What do you do beyond prescribing him the correct medication?

245. A 15-year old girl with a two-year-old child presents with a broken arm and requires surgery. The 15-year-old's guardian is not available to consent for the surgery. What do you do?

L. Informed Consent

246. A three-year-old female arrives in your emergency department unresponsive and with unstable vital signs. There is no adult available to consent for life-saving treatment. What do you do?

247. As a medical student, you are asked to consent an elderly woman for a hernia repair. She can barely hear and you are fairly confident she didn't understand the consent. When you tell the senior resident of your issue, she says, "Just get it done." What do you do?

248. Your patient requires gallbladder surgery and speaks only Thai. You do not speak Thai, and there are no interpreters available in the hospital. What do you do?

M. Medical Errors

249. How do you think we can decrease medical errors?

250. Do you think the US should have a national medical errors database? Why or why not?

251. Medical mistakes are common but not always important. Significant errors leading to morbidity, such as leaving a sponge in the abdomen after surgery, must be disclosed to patients. Should physicians also disclose less important mistakes, such a single inconsequential medication error?

252. What do you think about the current state of malpractice in the US?

N. Research Ethics

253. You are a fourth-year resident performing research and preparing to present your data at an upcoming global conference. Just before you leave, you discover your principal investigator (PI) is falsifying data. What do you do?

254. Many IRBs stipulate that researchers in developing countries provide the same standard of care for patients as they do in the US. What do you think about this stipulation?

255. If you could go back in time and ask Henrietta Lacks for permission to use her cells, would you?

O. Resource Allocation

256. Do you think healthcare should be rationed?

257. What if while you are spending more time with a terminally-ill elderly patient, you spend less time with a sick child, miss a diagnosis, and the child dies?

258. If you had $100,000 that could support one cancer patient or 100 healthy patients, how would you allocate the funds?

259. Of a seven-year-old girl with Down Syndrome, a 35-year-old single man with a former drug addiction, and a 51-year-old man with a wife and two children, to whom would you give a heart if you only had one?

260. I am the governor, and my wife wants to spend millions on an anti-meth campaign. What do you think about this use of funds?

P. Scientific Advancements

261. What do you think about genetic testing for [insert disease name]? (assume non-curable, life-threatening disease)?

262. How do you feel about stem cell research?

263. How do you feel advancements in gene therapy will affect the future of medicine?

264. What do you think about cloning?

Q. HIV and AIDS

265. Would you operate on a HIV+ patient that requires a minor knee operation?

266. Should we mandate HIV testing?

267. Do you think money is better spent researching HIV/AIDS treatment or cancer treatment?

XXI. Group

268. You three have just moved into a one-bedroom apartment together. Take 10 minutes to plan out how you are going to live with each other.

269.	If you were crashed on a desert island with a group of natives who worship wooden idols, and the pilot has a broken leg that is bleeding, what 5 items that are common to luggage would you want to have and why?
270.	Create a reality show where the winner gets a full ride to medical school.
271.	If you were the head of so and so company and we gave you 100 billion dollars, how would you allocate the money?
272.	You are on the organ transplant committee and have to choose between two individuals with liver damage who will die if they don't receive a new liver a) A 35-year-old mother with three children all below the age of 6 and a history of drug abuse b) A 50-year-old man with 20-year-old twins and a history of alcohol abuse. This person's family has given large donations to the school.
273.	A fourth-year medical student close to graduation messes up (ethically). What would you do to discipline him?
274.	A small town has a sudden surge in DUI and alcohol-related arrests. How would you go about researching the root of the problem?

It is natural to feel overwhelmed by this list. But by reading this book over the next seven weeks, performing the research and question practice suggested, and doing as many mock interviews as you can, you will be well-prepared for anything a medical school interviewer throws at you.

I'd like you to take the rest of this week to think about the questions just presented. Tomorrow, read the first question in each category and try to answer it out loud. No need to critique yourself yet. Just get comfortable answering a question out loud. The next day, pick another question from each of the 21 categories and answer it out loud. Then put the book down and take a break.

Next week, we'll start working through the first few categories. You will quickly see patterns develop and learn how to answer each question category with confidence.

WEEK 2

In Week 2, we will cover the most common question asked in all medical school interviews (can you guess what it is?), strategize how to handle the "Tell me about yourself" opening query, and review questions surrounding the nuts and bolts of your application. I suggest reading each chapter in full, and then brainstorming each question, practicing out loud as you go. This holds true for every question-and-answer-oriented chapter in the book, unless otherwise noted.

Day 1
Read Chapter 6 (Category I: Motivation for Medicine)
Brainstorm answers to questions

Day 2
Read Chapter 6 again
Review and revise initial brainstorming session
Practice answering each question out loud

Day 3
Read Chapter 7 (Category II: Open-ended)
Brainstorm answers to questions
Practice answering each question out loud

Day 4
Read Chapter 8 (Category III: Academics)
Brainstorm answers to questions
Practice answering each question out loud

Day 5
Read Chapter 9 (Category IV: Research)
Brainstorm answers to questions
Practice answering each question out loud

Day 6
Read Chapter 10 (Category V: Service) and Read Chapter 11 (Category VI: Extracurricular/Well-rounded)
Brainstorm answers to questions
Practice answering each question out loud

Day 7
Review Chapters 6-11
Practice motivation for medicine questions again
Practice any other questions you found challenging

CHAPTER 6

Category I: Motivation for Medicine

As proven by the AAMC survey of medical school admissions committees, motivation to enter medicine is the number one quality interviewers aim to assess in applicants. You will be asked about why you want to be a physician in some way in every interview. It really is "the" question, isn't it? Motivation for medicine questions are asked so often, it's easy to get bored with your own answer on the interview trail. But fight off this feeling. You want the answer to sound natural and compelling, even the fifth time you give it.

Go ahead and try to answer the question, "Why do you want to be a doctor?" in about 60 seconds. Harder than it seems, isn't it? Perhaps you started off with something like, "I want to enter medicine because I gain great satisfaction from helping others, and I love science." This is the most typical answer provided by pre-meds when first asked to describe their motivation for entering medicine. And it makes sense. Every future physician should want to help others and enjoy science, and most medical school interviewers assume you have these motivations as a starting point. But to stand out in medical school interviews, you must dive deeper than, "I like helping people, and I like science."

I suggest coming up with three talking points, as humans think best in groups of three. Remember this "rule of threes." You can use it often when answering medical school interview questions. Tie three talking points to concise personal anecdotes to help the interviewer remember your reasons. Why anecdotes? There is a scientific reason you likely already know. The hippocampus (memory) is connected to the amygdala (emotion). This is why we remember emotional events more easily than dull ones. This is also the reason incorporating cues that evoke emotion, such as humor, into study techniques improves memory and learning. The same is true of interviewers. After interviewing dozens of applicants, which will a medical school interviewer remember more easily – the name of a pre-med's community service project or that the project involved bushwhacking through the jungle to reach remote southeast Asian villages and deliver medical supplies? Use brief stories to help the interviewer remember you.

Here are some examples of how talking points can be tied to brief anecdotes to effectively answer "why medicine" questions. Use these examples to stimulate your own brainstorming process. Note how the rule of threes is stated explicitly in the first answer. Though it may feel awkward at first, it is very helpful to provide the interviewer with an opening sentence that tells her where the answer is going. It's similar to the thesis statement in essay writing. Providing a roadmap makes it easier for an interviewer to stay focused on your answer.

1. "Though there are many reasons I want to become a doctor, three stand out. First, I want to enter a profession where I work with others to solve life-altering problems every day. As a member of a clinical research team studying the effects of a new drug on lung cancer patients, I have seen the power of teamwork to make a direct impact on the lives of those who are ill. Further, I want to be a leader.

The medical hierarchy puts physicians as the default head of the medical team, and I look forward to using the skills gained as captain of the varsity swim team to lead effective teams, whether in the clinic or hospital. Finally, medicine will allow me to make an impact on related fields, such as health policy. After spending a gap year working with the Health Policy Institute, I have seen first hand how practicing clinicians are able to use their expertise to ensure health policy is created in light of the real world problems doctors and patients face everyday."

2. "I am drawn to the medical field because it lies at the intersection of art and science. As an avid reader and writer, I look forward to the story-telling aspect of doctoring, where exceptional history-taking and listening skills are used to unlock the scientific mystery at the core of any patient narrative. While shadowing Dr. Brown, an internist, I received a piece of advice I hope to use as the foundation of my medical practice. He said that a patient's history provides 90% of the information required to make an effective diagnosis and treatment plan. I have seen this maxim in action while volunteering at University Children's Hospital and during a medical mission trip to Nicaragua. I look forward to listening to my patients' stories and one day sharing these narratives through medical writing. I have already chronicled my experiences volunteering at the children's hospital through a weekly column in my university's newspaper."

3. "I want a career that allows me to work with individuals from all walks of life on a daily basis, encourages continual learning, and permits collaboration with other fields

including business and information technology. I love meeting new people and hearing about their lives. As a Spanish interpreter at Clinica Somos Hermanos in Los Angeles, I have enjoyed interacting with the patients, mostly undocumented immigrants, and hearing their harrowing stories of survival under harsh circumstances. Further, I religiously read the *New England Journal of Medicine* and look forward to a career with frequent advances and changes in standard practice – I know I will never be bored! Finally, as a self-taught programmer, I am drawn to medicine because it will allow me the ability to merge my interests in business and technology.

4. "My passion for medicine comes from a desire to bring cutting-edge laboratory work to the bedside. While working in Dr. Green's lab studying the possible uses of RNAi technology to treat Huntington's disease, I have met multiple patients with this devastating illness and have seen the impact such conditions have on both patients and family members. This experience fueled my desire to help create cures for conditions that are now incurable. But working in a lab is not enough for me. Volunteering at a local hospice and shadowing dozens of physicians have confirmed my desire to develop deep relationships with patients through a longitudinal practice. My dream is to become an academic neurologist who runs both a clinic and basic science laboratory, so I can help patients individually and use research to create solutions to help larger populations."

5. "I am drawn to the medical field because I want to become a surgeon who uses teamwork, hand-eye coordination, and advanced technology to make a tangible impact on the lives

of others both in the US and abroad. As a theater director in college, I have enjoyed bringing disparate people together to create a powerful production. I hope to use my skills as a physician to lead effective teams directly caring for others. I also look forward to using my brain and hands to solve problems. I have been an avid tinkerer since age 10, when I disassembled the family piano and then reassembled it, and love using my manual skills to fix and create things. I am also a technophile, and like how medicine, particularly surgery, is on the pulse of cutting edge technology. In addition to my US-based practice, I am interested in setting up mobile surgical clinics in developing nations. I have spent the last three summers working for Hospital Ships in an administrative role and have witnessed the remarkable impact surgeons have in underserved areas."

Now let's walk through the list of questions under the motivation for medicine category and see how the answer created from the brainstorming exercise can be adapted to each question.

Please note Q = Question and A = Answer throughout the rest of the book.

Q1: *Why do you want to be a doctor?*
A1: Give the "why medicine" answer you prepared through the brainstorming exercise.

Q2: *When did you first become interested in medicine?*
A2: You have two options here:

1. Provide an anecdote about the first time you felt an interest in medicine if you had such an experience. Move quickly to how you have further investigated the field

and confirmed it is the "right profession for me for the following reasons...." Then give the reasons you prepared for the "why medicine" answer. You may have to shorten your original "why medicine" answer to prevent rambling. Given we 21st century humans have an ever-shortening attention span, I suggest keeping most answers to about 60 seconds or less whenever possible. If you must go longer, definitely keep your answer to less than 90 seconds.

2. State there was not a clear time when you first became interested in medicine because it was more of a gradual reckoning. Then give the reasons prepared for the "why medicine" answer.

Q3: *Did you have an "aha" moment when you decided medicine was the career for you?*

A3: Employ the same strategy as used to answer Q2. Isn't it great when the same answer can be used for multiple questions?

Q4: *Why doctor and not PA, NP, or RN?*

A4: Hopefully, your "why medicine" answer already includes reasons that imply why MD as opposed to physician assistant, nurse practitioner, or nurse. If not, create one more reason that differentiates the MD from the other fields. Common reasons refer to differing leadership roles, responsibilities, decision-making techniques, and training. Be careful never to put down the other professions. Instead, praise the MD role and explain why it is right for you.

Q5: *I see your father/mother is a doctor. Prove to me you are not going into medicine to please him/her/them.*

A5: On the surface, this seems like a harsh question. But it is often what interviewers are thinking because so many children of doctors want to become doctors. Again, you can reuse the "why medicine" answer as it will show you understand the field thoroughly and have made your own decision. But instead of immediately launching into your prepared "why medicine" answer, I suggest you first address the question directly. For example, "Yes, my mother is a physician and listening to her speak about her job every night at the dinner table certainly peaked my interest in the field. But I have explored the profession thoroughly and want to enter it for the following reasons." Then give a version of the "why medicine" answer.

Q6: *I understand there are no/few doctors in your family. How do you know it's the right profession for you?*

A6: If this question pertains to you, take the same strategy as suggested for the "prove you are not going into medicine to please your parents" question. Start with an opening line, such as, "You are correct, there are no doctors in my immediate family. But I have explored the profession thoroughly and want to enter it for the following reasons." Then give a version of the "why medicine" answer. Do you see how a pattern is forming? Use an opening sentence to directly address the question, and then adapt the "why medicine" answer to provide more depth.

Q7: *What do you hope to get out of medicine?*

A7: Isn't this question really asking about your reasons for entering medicine? Let's say your "why medicine" answer is the first example provided in the brainstorming exercise above. You can easily modify it to discuss your hopes for a medical career. For example,

"I hope to get a few things out of medicine. I want to feel the satisfaction of working with others to solve life-altering problems every day as I did as a member of clinical research team studying the effects of a new drug on lung cancer patients. Further, I hope to be a leader who uses the skills I learned in the pool to guide effective teams. Finally, I want to make an impact in the field of health policy. After spending a gap year working with the Health Policy Institute, I have seen first hand how practicing clinicians are able to use their expertise to ensure health policy is created in light of the real world problems doctors and patients face everyday."

Notice how the same three reasons are given but with a few tweaks to answer the specific question. It is possible, though unlikely, you will be asked both the "why do you want to be a doctor" and the "what do you hope to get out of medicine" questions. If this is the case, you can reiterate the "why medicine" answer quickly, and then provide a few more specifics about what you hope medicine will provide you. For example, you may want to gain satisfaction from helping others daily, learn something new every day, or be part of a field with links to business and policy.

Q8:   *Has anyone attempted to dissuade you from becoming a physician? If so, how did you respond?*

A8:   This is becoming a common question given all of the current problems facing healthcare in the US. This question is really asking, "Do you know what you are getting yourself into?" Even if no one has directly attempted to dissuade you from becoming a doctor, you have to provide an answer showing the interviewer you understand the problems facing healthcare today. But, as with all negative questions, you want to refocus the question to the positive quickly and discuss why you do

67

want to enter the field. Here's how, using "why medicine" answer example #3:

"Multiple physicians I have shadowed or worked with at the free clinic have spoken to me about the difficult parts of their jobs, such as endless paperwork, insurance hassles, and the general stress of caring for sick people. One even said to me, 'Do you really want to get yourself into this mess?' After exploring the field through shadowing, clinical volunteering, and clinical research, my response to such questions has been that, in my opinion, the positives outweigh the negatives."

Then incorporate your "why medicine" answer:

"I want a career that allows me to work with individuals from all walks of life on a daily basis, encourages continual learning, and permits collaboration with other fields including business and information technology. That career is medicine."

Q9: *If you could not be a doctor, what would you do?*

A9: Ugh, another negative question. But that's ok, because now you know how to refocus a negative to a positive. It's not good enough to say something like, "This is the only profession for me," but you can begin by reaffirming your interest in medicine. Then use your "why medicine" reasons to answer the question. Here's an example of how to modify "why medicine" answer example #4:

"Given my passion for medicine comes from a desire to bring cutting-edge laboratory work to the bedside, I think my skills would be best used as a physician-researcher. If this path was closed to me, I guess I would pursue research while trying to keep my hand in the clinical side of medicine wherever possible. This would be far from ideal, however, as I have seen while working in Dr. Green's lab studying the possible uses of RNAi technology to treat Huntington's disease. Here I have learned how obtaining a physician's education and bedside experience is a key to making the biggest contribution in the field."

Look at that! Nine common medical school interview questions answered by modifying one response. Your answers to these motivation for medicine questions are so important that I suggest you put the book down for today, do a brainstorming session, and practice out loud. Then re-read this chapter again tomorrow. After you have re-read it, review your brainstorming and again practice answering each question out loud. Even better, record yourself on video and then watch the recording with a critical eye. It will be painful to watch and listen to yourself at first, but it will get easier with time. Other than doing mock interviews with an admissions expert, watching yourself on video is the best way to practice.

CHAPTER 7

Category II: Open-ended

Though it is a bit of a lazy way to begin an interview, many interviewers will start with an open-ended question. If you haven't prepared for such a question, it can be difficult to know how to answer. But instead of thinking of them as a burden, view open-ended questions as an opportunity because they give you the ability to guide the interview tone and topics.

Q10: *Tell me about yourself.*

A10: Although it would take days to answer this question in depth, you have about 60 seconds to describe aspects of yourself that will pique the interviewer's interest and serve as a springboard to further questions and conversation. I suggest giving a broad overview of your life, starting with childhood, breezing through high school years, and ending with college/post-college life, all while highlighting major milestones you think make you standout. Here's how I would have answered this question as a pre-med:

"I was born and raised in the suburbs of Washington, DC, where, as the third and youngest daughter in the family, I was quite outgoing and adventurous. My mother, an English and drama teacher, found me performing my balance beam routine on the yellow double lines in the middle of our street when I was two. My father, an aerospace engineer, is a huge sports fan and harnessed my energy by ensuring a ball was in my hand as much as possible. I remember my childhood fondly. I filled my free time with soccer and basketball tournaments and swim meets. I attended a local junior high and high school and had the privilege of traveling the country through athletics. I was first introduced to medicine when a teammate playing next to me tore her ACL during a national championship game junior year. Watching her treatment and recovery triggered an interest in medicine and exploration of the field through hospital shadowing and volunteering. I then attended Harvard, where I majored in History and Science, took pre-med classes as electives, and played basketball for all four years, becoming captain senior year. After graduation, I joined the Institute of Medicine as a research assistant, where I am currently working on medical error and immunization finance reports."

A chronological answer interspersed with interesting details provides the interviewer with many possible follow-up questions.

Q11: What was your childhood like?

A11: You can respond to this question by using the beginning of your "tell me about yourself" answer, which focuses on your childhood, and adding a few more details. Remember, short anecdotes recounting interesting times in your childhood (such as pretending the street lines were a balance beam) will help the interviewer remember you.

Q12: *Tell me about your family/upbringing.*

A12: Again, you can adapt the beginning of the "tell me about yourself" answer to easily answer this question.

Q13: *What would you like me to know?*

A13: I view this question as slightly different from the "tell me about yourself" type of open-ended questions. It is so broad, I suggest providing a more specific answer and, instead of giving your life story, answer with two to three interesting facts about yourself. These facts can highlight the most significant parts of your application, update the interviewer on a recent activity, and/or provide interesting information not included on the application. Like all open-ended questions, "what would you like me to know" is putting you in the interview driver's seat. Whatever topics you bring up will likely set the tone for the rest of the interview.

Don't feel the need to discuss only medically-related topics in your answer. If the interviewer wants to know specifically about your motivation for medicine or another part of your application, she will ask. When trying to pick topics for this answer, think about what you love to talk about, what you are most proud of not already on your application, and what aspects of your life make you stand out.

Q14: *Tell me something I can't find anywhere on your application.*

A14: You may have created an answer to this question by preparing for your "what would you like me to know" response. You can talk about anything from hobbies to the latest book you read to interesting family history. Again, consider your passions, sources of pride, and unique life experiences. Feel free to think outside the box and devise an answer that will make the interviewer sit up and say, "Tell me more about that."

Q15: *What is one question you wish we had asked you? Please answer it.*

A15: Though packaged in a creative form, this is just another way of asking you to tell the interviewer something new about yourself. Through your open-ended interview preparation, answering this question will be a breeze because you already have multiple interesting facts about yourself ready to discuss.

You can take an alternative approach to this question and use it to provide information you believe is critical to your application but has not yet been discussed in the interview. If you take this angle, you can use answers prepared for other common topics, such as research and community service experiences.

Q16: *Is there anything else you would like me to know?*

A16: Along with, "do you have any questions for me?" the "anything else you would like me to know?" question is the most common last query in a medical school interview. Though many pre-meds answer, "I don't think so," I strongly suggest you have a specific answer ready. Quickly think back over what topics were discussed in the interview. If there are any strengths of your application that did not come up, now is the time to raise them. If the interview has already touched on all of your application highlights, use one of the interesting facts you planned for a "what would you like me to know?" type of open-ended question. There is no need to ramble on in order to keep the interview session going. Provide a short and interesting response and see if the interviewer wants to engage further or say goodbye.

Now take time to brainstorm answers to Chapter 7 questions and practice out loud.

CHAPTER 8

Category III: Academics

Many interviewers, especially those in a closed file interview, will want to chat about your academic background. The questions in the academic category are, thankfully, relatively straightforward. Most interviewers are not trying to trip you up, but instead want to gain a sense of how you have made academic choices. The vast majority of medical school interviewers have no interest in whether you know the details of ATP phosphorylation or DNA synthesis. Such content knowledge is assessed in your academic transcript and MCAT score. Academic questions focus more on motivation, breadth, and well-roundedness. Remember, even if you are many years out of undergrad, all college courses and experiences are fair game.

Q17: *Why did you choose your undergraduate institution?*

A17: This clear-cut question requires a clear-cut answer. In your response, you can use the rule of three to provide three main reasons why you chose to attend a certain college. I hope it is obvious you want to refrain from including reasons such as, "I was looking for a party school," or, "I didn't do well in high school and Mediocre College was the only place I was accepted." As with all interview question answers, you want your reasons to reflect positively on yourself.

Q18: Why did you choose your undergraduate major?

A18: Another straightforward question. Describe to the interviewer what drew you to your field of choice. If you are/were a humanities major, there is no need to apologize for not majoring in science. In fact, medical school admissions committees tend to favor humanities majors, as they are usually well-rounded students nurturing the right side of the brain.

Q19: What was your favorite college course and why?

A19: This is a fun question because you can discuss a course you found inspiring. And when interviewees discuss something truly inspiring, it is easy to show passion without appearing forced. You don't have to pick a science or medically-related course. A theme is forming here – medical schools appreciate well-rounded applicants. This is why "pre-med" is not a major, but just a set of 12, one-semester courses. These requirements leave ample time to explore a range of topics. Medical schools want applicants who have broad academic interests.

Q20: What was your least favorite college course and why?

A20: What do we do with negative questions? Refocus them to the positive as quickly as possible. The best way to answer this query is to describe a course where you initially struggled for some reason (difficult material, notorious instructor, *etc.*), but overcame the initial difficulties to master the material. Answers to negative questions usually should be short. This is a good tactic because you want to move along to other more positive questions quickly.

Q21: What class impressed you the most positively or negatively in your undergraduate education?

A21: It will come as no surprise to you that I suggest answering the "positively" part of this question. Fortunately, you already have answers created for both sides of this query based on preparation of Q19 and Q20.

Q22: *Do you feel your undergraduate education has challenged you?*
A22: The "no-duh" initial answer is an emphatic, "Yes." But then you must support this answer with specifics from your undergraduate experience. An anecdote or two will suffice.

Q23: *Describe your undergraduate education.*
A23: This is an open-ended question you may take in any direction you please. Of course, keep it as positive as possible. And be sure to include important specifics such as how you chose your school and major and what courses inspired you. Don't feel pigeonholed into only discussing academics alone. "Education" often occurs outside of the classroom.

Q24: *What is your greatest academic achievement?*
A24: Many pre-meds cite typical academic achievements, such as winning scholarships, grants, and awards; writing a thesis; or succeeding in a particularly difficult class. These answers are perfectly acceptable. But you don't have to draw your answer from inside of the classroom. "Academics" can be viewed broadly and defined as any intellectual pursuit. Feel free to use achievements, such as research, that occurred through extracurriculars.

Q25: *Are you a crammer or do you study a little each day?*
A25: When answering this question about your study habits, be honest. Though many argue "cramming" is less effective than studying a bit each day, there is no right way to study. You

may honestly describe how you study and perhaps discuss the evolution of your study habits, especially if you struggled academically at some point.

Q26: *In what environment do you learn best?*

A26: With most medical schools in the US moving to problem-based learning (PBL), medical school admissions committees want to ensure you will learn well in a cooperative environment. Though, of course, you want to give an honest answer to this (and all) questions, it's important to understand the motivation behind common queries in the medical school interview. Prior to coming to an interview, you will have researched the school's curriculum. Use this information to help mold your answer and highlight a part of the specific medical school's curriculum that matches your learning style.

Q27: *What was something you learned for fun?*

A27: I love this question because it allows you to show you understand how learning doesn't happen just inside a formal classroom. Your answer can highlight fun parts of your application, such a hobbies and side interests. Answers to these types of questions often lead to the most engaging discussions in medical school interviews.

Q28: *How did your study abroad experience affect you and your studies?*

A28: There is a growing belief that study abroad experiences are filled with mostly play and little academic rigor. When answering such a question, focus on what you learned both inside and outside of the classroom understanding the interviewer may be skeptical of the benefits of studying abroad. It is your job to convince the interviewer of the positives of the experience beyond the sexiness of travel.

Q29: Why did you obtain a graduate degree?

A29: If you have pursued graduate studies, many interviewers will want to know your motivation. This is the perfect time to use the rule of three to provide three reasons you decided to continue your studies. Remember to connect these reasons to interesting anecdotes.

Q30: Tell me about your graduate studies.

A30: Another open-ended question. I suggest starting with your motivation for going to graduate school (*i.e.*, the answer you have prepared for Q29), providing a brief description of your course of study, and concluding with what you gained from the experience.

It's brainstorm and response time. Hopefully Chapter 8's questions will be relatively easy for you to answer. And remember to practice out loud (and record yourself if possible).

CHAPTER 9

Category IV: Research

Research is a common topic in medical school interviews, even if you are not pursuing the MD/PhD route. Generally, research questions are not particularly tricky. Interviewers are usually more interested in the overall research hypothesis and significance of the results than in the intricacies of your exact lab or project role. One of the biggest mistakes I have seen pre-meds make when preparing for research questions is spending too much time on the minutiae of their DNA splicing tasks or SAS stats run while spending too little time on how their specific tasks fit into the larger goals of the lab or project. It is critical to know how all the investigation parts fit together, especially if your study has been published. For example, it's not good enough to say, "I didn't do the stats" or, "I wasn't part of the lab when the methodology was created" when asked about the statistics or methods of the paper, respectively. Be sure to understand the entire project, whether you were part of the study for one summer or four years.

Q31: *Tell me about your research.*

A31: All scientists, including physicians, are taught to think about research in the standardized abstract form, sometimes referred to as IMRaD:

Introduction
Methods
Results
Discussion

Doctors become so attuned to thinking about research in IMRaD form that listening to a pre-med describe research in any other way can be difficult. Whenever discussing your research, use the abstract form. It will make both giving and receiving the answer easier.

When following the abstract form, guard against speaking for longer than a minute. Ideally, answers should be less than 60 seconds. By hitting the highlights, the interviewer will understand the most important parts of your research and may ask follow-up questions as he desires.

Here are some examples of abstract form answers for different types of research (because, of course, all research does not occur in the lab). I have inserted the abstract parts in parenthesis to show you how to present in IMRaD. You don't have to state these words in your answer.

1. (Introduction) I have worked at the Best Laboratory at The University for the last two years studying the basic science of protease inhibitors in hepatitis C treatment. (Methods) Our methods involve using rat models infected with different strains of hepatitis C to investigate how the same protease inhibitor affects viral load in each type of infection. (Results) Preliminary results show the protease inhibitor in question decreases viral load in each type of infection by at least 50%, but has a differing impact based on exact viral strain. Fortunately, there appear to be few side effects experienced by the rats. (Discussion) This research is important for two reasons. First, it shows the protease

inhibitor used in the study decreases viral load in hepatitis C-infected rats with few side effects. We hope such results will be repeated in humans in future studies. Second, it demonstrates differing impact of the drug on differing hepatitis C strains. We expect to have definitive findings ready for publication in the next six months.

2. (Introduction) I have had multiple research experiences in the last four years, but would like to tell you about the one I have found most impactful. For the past year, I have worked at the Institute of Science as a research assistant on a project studying medical errors in tertiary referral centers in the United States. (Methods) We targeted the largest, by patient volume, tertiary referral centers in each of the 50 states and implemented an anonymous medical errors database system in each hospital to record medical error events over a three-year period. (Results) We are currently in the third year of data collection. Though the data has not been collected in full, we are already seeing patterns in medical errors involving certain types of drugs and specific times of day, such as shift change. (Discussion) We expect to publish full results in just over a year. By understanding what errors occur and when, we hope the study will serve as a springboard for medical error prevention programs.

3. (Introduction) My research has involved working with clinicians and engineers to develop a portable, cost-effective, and simple-to-use hemoglobin monitor for use the developing world. Millions of developing-world residents suffer from preventable anemia, a major risk factor for lethal postpartum hemorrhage. The most common laboratory machine to diagnose anemia costs

$10,000 and requires a trained technician – resources not available in many developing world locations. (Methods) Using technology similar to pulse oximetry, we have developed an inexpensive, portable hemoglobin monitor run on two AA batteries and easily used by community health workers. (Results) We have rolled out the device in over 1,000 rural clinics in India and have partnered with a local university to perform effectiveness studies looking at anemia rates and postpartum hemorrhage incidence. (Discussion) We believe this product will dramatically reduce the prevalence of preventable anemia by allowing easy diagnosis. Fortunately, treatment for anemia with iron and/or folic acid is inexpensive and generally available in even the most resource-limited environments.

Q32: *What research have you done and why?*

A32: The only difference between this question and Q31 is the "and why?" You can modify your prepared answer in abstract form by either beginning or ending with your motivation for pursuing the research.

Q33: *What is the most impactful research you have done?*

A33: Yah! Another question you can repeat a previously prepared answer.

Q34: *Pretend you are at a conference presenting your most important research, and I am in the audience. Give me your presentation.*

A34: Guess what? Conference presentations almost always follow abstract form! Simply give your prepared research answer.

Q35: *Do you expect to continue performing research during medical school?*

A35: If you do expect to continue research in medical school, this answer is easy. Describe your future research goals and try to tie in details regarding how the school where you are interviewing will help you accomplish these goals because of specific laboratory, course, or research opportunities available there. If you have no interest in pursuing research in medical school, the answer can be trickier. The key is to quickly explain why you do not expect to continue with research, and then move on to how you will fill the time in other interesting ways. For example,

> "Though I gained valuable lessons in patience and teamwork when working in Blues Laboratory, I often found myself daydreaming about how I could be spending the time more directly assisting patients. I certainly expect to be a physician who stays up-to-date on the latest research but prefer to spend my time at the bedside rather than in the lab. In medical school, I expect to use my free time to work in the Uninsured Clinic. That being said, I would be happy to get involved in clinical research in the future, as long as the investigation involves working directly with patients."

Q36: *What labs or research institutions at this school particularly interest you?*

A36: Because you have already researched the school thoroughly, it will be easy for you to roll out two or three research opportunities of interest to you. You want to be as specific as possible in this answer. Name labs, professors, institutions, groups, *etc.*, as opposed to simply mentioning a genre of research you want to perform.

Q37: *Tell me about your publications.*

A37: If you have publications, present them in abstract form, which should now be second nature to you. If you have an abstract or conference presentation, provide details of it. If you have no publications, abstracts, or presentations, state this matter of factly and then segway into the research you have performed, assuming you have not already discussed it. And remember, you can discuss your contribution to research included in a publication even if you are not named as an author. You can also discuss future plans to publish.

Being part of a publication in a peer-reviewed journal is not a requirement of any MD program in the US, so don't feel defeated by this question if you have not published. Refocus the answer to the positive and discuss future goals. Of course, MD/PhD programs have a higher research bar and often expect candidates to have publications under their belt.

Q38: *Why is your research not published?*

A38: Ouch. This is a tough question, but one for which you must be prepared. Go through each research experience that has not resulted in a publication and brainstorm why. There are many legitimate possible answers including the research is not complete, the study results are not statistically significant and it is difficult to get negative results published, the research has been submitted for publication and you are waiting to hear from the journal, the research has been submitted for publication and rejected (give reasons for rejection), or their were fatal flaws in the research making the results unusable.

As with any challenging questions, do not show offense. Smile and give your answer in a non-defensive way. It is very hard to get published, and, as I said previously, having a publication is not a requirement of MD schools. If you provide sound reasons for lack of publication and show you understand the details of how research really works, even the harshest interviewer will be impressed.

Q39: *If you were given a $1 million grant to perform research, what would you do with it?*

A39: Many pre-meds cringe at these "creative" questions. But you should learn to love them. Such queries provide an opportunity to think outside the box and dream big. Expand research you are currently performing, start a novel investigation, or enter a new field. Strong answers to this question occur when pre-meds follow their passions.

We've reached the end of Chapter 9, which means it's time to brainstorm and practice. Don't hesitate to pull out your research notes, poster presentations, abstracts, or publications to ensure you understand the research at the necessary level of detail. You may even want to schedule a meeting with previous research colleagues to discuss specifics if they are unclear to you. Investigate your research!

CHAPTER 10

Category V: Service

Medicine is a service profession. As such, many interviewers will try to assess your desire to serve others, both in a medical setting and in the greater community. In addition, many medical schools include service to disadvantaged or at-risk communities as a core part of their mission and want to ensure their future medical students share this passion.

Q40: *How have you served the community?*

A40: Start answering this question by listing all of your service experiences. For example, "I have served the community in many ways, including teaching science to underprivileged children, running a fundraiser for the last four years for Relay for Life, volunteering in a free clinic and hospital, and traveling to Peru on a medical mission." Then describe in more detail the experience you found most meaningful or impactful. For example, "I'd like to tell you more about the medical mission to Peru, as I found it the most impactful because..." Continue with a brief description of the experience.

As you have read in this book many times, every answer does not need to directly relate to medicine. Sometimes highlighting a non-medical experience showing you possess characteristics directly applicable to medicine, such as empathy, leadership, and teaching skills, will make you stand out.

Q41: What was your most meaningful community service experience?

A41: You prepared the answer to this question is your response to Q40. See how much easier preparation becomes when questions are broken down into categories?

Q42: Do you think your volunteer work makes a real difference?

A42: Such cynical questions can be answered easily with the truth – of course you think your volunteer work makes a real difference for yourself and the individuals or communities you serve. Don't be shocked by such negative questions. Keep your poise and create a positive answer supported by your experience. And remember, you don't have to find the cure for cancer or save starving children in Africa to make a difference. Small gestures, such as reading to lonely nursing home residents or taking your little buddy to a sporting event, can be just as impactful.

Q43: Describe a specific time you helped someone in the last two weeks.

A43: It's hard to have a standard answer to this question for every interview because your interview dates could be separated by months. But do think about how you would answer this question now. By doing so, you will be more prepared to think of an answer quickly on the interview day. Once again remember "helping" can have a broad meaning. Don't immediately pigeon-hole yourself into a medically-related answer. To get your creative juices flowing, here are some examples you may not have thought of immediately but certainly fit the "helping" category:

- Tutored a colleague
- Babysat your sister
- Gave a friend a ride
- Lent your brother money
- Bought lunch for a homeless man
- Let your roommate borrow your bike◎
- Carried groceries for an elderly neighbor
- Baked cookies to cheer up a friend
- Sent a surprise gift to your niece
- Mowed your parents' lawn while they were out of town
- Taught a non-techy older man how to use an iPhone
- Helped your classmate prepare for the medical school interview
- Took notes for a friend who missed class due to illness
- Sent articles to your cousin to encourage interest in science
- Stayed late at the lab to help post-doc with an experiment

Q44: *Tell me about your service trip abroad.*

A44: An increasing number of pre-meds are joining medical or other service teams who travel abroad to provide care or assistance. If you have done so, describe the teams' goals, your role, and what you gained from the experience. Don't worry if you haven't traveled abroad for a service trip, as it is unlikely you will be asked this question unless such an experience has been included on your application.

Q45: *Do you really think a two-week service trip made a real difference to the community you served?*

A45: Wow. Another cynical question, but one I think is important. More and more, Western-based medical and other service teams raise money and travel to low-resource environments to provide short-term care. It is only natural for the question to arise: "Does two weeks have an impact?" For many trips, such as those providing surgical services or helping implement clean water or irrigation systems, the answer is an easily supported, "Yes." For others, the impact might be more difficult to define. Think deeply about your trip and the impact it made. Then answer honestly.

If you feel the trip did not make the impact you had hoped, feel comfortable being honest. Some of the best interviews I have held stemmed from pre-meds providing a truthful assessment of an experience that did not meet expectations, and then discussing how the experience could be improved in the future. Reflecting on mistakes or less-than-stellar experiences and providing information on improvement opportunities (remember, refocus to the positive!) shows a maturity many medical school admissions committees are seeking in candidates.

Q46: *Is medicine a service profession?*

A46: Of course it is. That's the easy part of the answer. Now you have to defend why medicine as a service profession. Provide personal experience(s) in the medical setting as evidence for your opinions. For example,

> "I can't think of a profession that is more based in service. While volunteering at St. Luke's Hospital, I saw evidence of doctors serving other's daily and not only when diagnosing a problem and providing treatment, but when offering hope after giving bad news, finding housing for a homeless patient about to be discharged, and stepping in to assist the team in tasks often relegated to the nursing staff, such as removing bed pans and taking vital signs."

Specific examples are the key to this answer. They will both help the interviewer remember you and also show your deep knowledge of how medicine really works.

As this was a short chapter, I suggest reading the next chapter (Chapter 11) as well, and then brainstorming and practicing your service and extracurricular questions together.

CHAPTER 11

Category VI: Extracurricular/ Well-rounded

As we've already discussed, medical school admissions committees are looking for well-rounded applicants. Extracurriculars, or how you spend your time outside of traditional academic pursuits, are often the best way to shine. Sometimes the majority of a medical school interview will involve discussion of a unique hobby or interest. It's so much more fun for an interviewer to learn about your bike collection, or recent trip to Borneo, or the fifth language you learned, or the painting you just completed than about your EMT training or pipetting in the lab. It's human nature to want to discuss what makes you different. So be ready to discuss how you spend your free time outside of typical pre-med pursuits and be proud of what you have accomplished.

Q47: *What do/did you spend most of your time doing outside the classroom?*

A47: This question presents the perfect opportunity to discuss the extracurricular activities that make you stand out. Anything goes here – from sports to arts to hobbies to languages to exotic travel. I suggest staying away from answers such as "Hanging out with friends" or "Studying." Even "Reading" or "Watching movies" are pretty boring answers. Let's say you really do spend most of your free time relaxing with friend or watching movies. Provide specifics to make these facts more interesting. For example, "I take great pride in forming deep friendships and being known as a good listener. Thus, I spend a lot of time outside the classroom meeting with friends, discussing their lives, and often helping work out any issues they are facing." Or you could say, "I find nothing more relaxing and enjoyable than watching a great movie. In fact, I've become a bit of a movie buff, studying my favorite directors – Wes Anderson and Francis Ford Coppola – and enrolling in a cinematography course at the local community college." Do you see how adding specifics makes the common activities of visiting friends and watching films so much more interesting?

Q48: *Tell me about your most meaningful extracurricular experience.*

A48: Pick the extracurricular you feel has made the most impact on either your life or the lives of others. Feel free to use the answer given to Q47 if you are able to explain why it is meaningful. Because anything goes for extracurriculars, feel free to talk about activities not directly related to medicine. You want to show your well-roundedness at any opportunity.

Q49: *What do you do for fun?*

A49: Another great question allowing you to be yourself, highlight your well-roundedness, and stand out. You can either use the prepared answer for "what do/did you spend most of your time doing outside the classroom?" or pick another topic entirely. Medical schools don't want a bunch of book worms that do nothing but study. They want students who have a life. Have fun with this "fun" question.

Q50: *What are your hobbies?*

A50: According to Oxford Dictionaries online (http://www. oxforddictionaries.com), a hobby is defined as:

> "noun" (plural hobbies)
>
> 1 an activity done regularly in one's leisure time for pleasure:
>
> her hobbies are reading and gardening
>
> 2 (archaic) a small horse or pony

Let's ignore the "small horse or pony" and focus on the first definition, which could be describing an extracurricular. Premeds often struggle with this question and tell me, "But I don't have any hobbies. I don't collect stamps or cook." They are taking a very narrow view of hobbies. Look at how you spend your free time, and I bet you will find some hobbies. Music, painting, exercising, learning martial arts, knitting, building a website/programming, studying a language, and playing cards/games can all be described as hobbies. Think broadly.

Q51: *Pretend you've been working and studying nonstop for weeks and you finally have a day off. What do you do with it?*

A51: Such a fun question! Don't think too hard about this one. Instead, use your gut answer, as it often the best one. The great thing about this query is the opportunity to show what you do to relax and have fun, which often says a lot about you.

Q52: *Why are you in a sorority/fraternity?*

A52: On the surface, this question seems to have a negative connotation. But don't take it that way. Many pre-meds are afraid to mention their involvement in their school's Greek system in any way, given the typical stereotype of such institutions as gateways to drunken rowdiness. However, many sororities and fraternities refute this stereotype and provide opportunities for service, leadership, and community. If you are in one of these types of sororities/fraternities, talk about your motivations and experiences with pride.

Q53: *Are you involved in the arts in any way?*

A53: If you are involved in the arts, describe your experience. You don't have to be Michelangelo or undertake formal study to say yes to this question. Painting or playing an instrument for stress relief, writing a blog on your favorite topic, or performing stand-up comedy for charity are all art forms worthy of discussion. If you have never been involved in any sort of art, state this fact then shift the answer to how you have spent your free time in other ways.

Q54: *Are you involved in sports?*

A54: You may answer this question in the affirmative even if you don't participate in Division I athletics. Experiences such as playing on club or intramural teams, exercising for health, managing a team, or cheering on your favorite team are all worthy of mention.

Q55: *What do you do for exercise?*

A55: Given you are about to enter a field that promotes regular exercise as one of the key components of a healthy lifestyle, you hopefully engage in some sort of exercise yourself. Once again, you don't have to be an Olympic athlete to create an interesting response to this question. Running/walking, playing pick-up sports, lifting weights, yoga, dancing, and martial arts are all forms of exercise, just to name a few. If you have a disability that prevents regular exercise, then of course you can answer no and explain.

I suggest brainstorming the questions covered in Chapters 10 and 11 now. Then give yourself a rest and return tomorrow to review Chapters 6-11. Be sure to practice the motivation for medicine questions again. And again and again. Then move on to any questions you found most challenging in Week 2.   Quick tip: if you found a certain question easy to answer and are confident in the strength of your response, don't waste time repeatedly practicing it. Put your effort into what is hard and needs improvement.

WEEK 3

W eek 3 questions will feel similar to your secondary essay prompts. Many pre-meds wonder if they need to come up with different answers for interview questions that repeat what is covered on the primary or secondary applications. There is no need to present new themes when asked similar questions over different parts of the application, but it is a good idea to provide new specifics. Let's say you are passionate about pubic health. It's great to speak about this passion in your personal statement, in response to the secondary essay prompt on future goals, and when asked in an interview about where you see yourself in 20 years. Just try to use different anecdotes to support your points in each essay or interview answer. Using the same details for each is too repetitive. But themes can and should be used over and over again.

Focus on a chapter per day for the first six days of this week, again brainstorming and answering questions out loud/ recording yourself as you go. Then use the final day to review the week and re-address the challenging questions.

Day 1
Read Chapter 12 (Category VII: Clinical Experience)
Brainstorm answers to questions
Practice answering each question out loud

Day 2
Read Chapter 13 (Category VIII: Application-related)

Brainstorm answers to questions
Practice answering each question out loud

Day 3
Read Chapter 14 (Category IX: Future)
Brainstorm answers to questions
Practice answering each question out loud

Day 4
Read Chapter 15 (Category X: Diversity)
Brainstorm answers to questions
Practice answering each question out loud

Day 5
Read Chapter 16 (Category XI: Coping Skills)
Brainstorm answers to questions
Practice answering each question out loud

Day 6
Read Chapter 17 (Category XII: Professionalism/Physician Role)
Brainstorm answers to questions
Practice answering each question out loud

Day 7
Review Chapters 12-17
Practice any questions you found challenging

CHAPTER **12**

Category VII: Clinical Experience

I cannot emphasize enough the importance of clinical experience to medical school admissions committees. Through clinical experience, you are able to prove to both yourself and admissions committees that you truly understand the day-to-day responsibilities of being a physician. Shadowing, observing, volunteering, and working in any clinical settings, such as hospitals, clinics, offices, nursing homes, hospices, and homes (homecare) of loved ones, are all beneficial clinical experiences you may draw upon to answer the following questions. Being a patient is also valid clinical experience.

Q56: Which clinical experience did you find most impactful?

A56: You can answer this question in the same way you answered other "most impactful" questions. Briefly state your multiple clinical experiences, and then identify the one you believe has been most impactful. For example, "I have volunteered in the emergency department, worked as an EMT, shadowed seven physicians, and played violin for residents in a nursing home. I found volunteering in the ED the most meaningful of these experiences." Then give details about the particular experience you have chosen to highlight. Many pre-meds feel they made little difference during their clinical time. I have two responses to such worries: First, you likely did make a difference, as even small gestures can be incredibly helpful in a medical setting, and second, you are not a doctor yet! Clinical experience is more about understanding the medical world and what you are getting into, rather than how great an impact you have made on others. Do not belittle your experiences.

Q57: *What was your most memorable physician shadowing experience?*

A57: Medical school admissions committees assume you have shadowed multiple physicians to gain an understanding of the breath of opportunities available in medicine. Responding to this question is your chance to highlight the most memorable experience. Many pre-meds jump to dramatic examples, such as observing CPR or an intricate surgery. But remember medicine is often more about the mundane than the spectacular. Don't shy away from discussing the little things doctors often do, such as remembering a patient's children, giving a hug, or providing education in the hope of changing a patient's behavior.

Q58: *Tell me about the most interesting case you have seen.*

A58: Pre-meds also like to answer this one with gory, intense, or extraordinary cases. Feel free to do so. But be aware "interesting" means different things to different people. I am always more impressed with the pre-meds who show they understand medicine doesn't have to be flashy by highlighting the importance of small gestures in helping others.

Q59: *Prove to me you know what it's like to be a doctor.*

A59: This blunt question encompasses what underlies all of the other clinical experience questions. You can prove you know what it's like to be a doctor by describing your clinical experience. This is a good question to answer by describing both the breadth and the depth of your clinical experience.

Q60: *Tell me about an experience during your shadowing that made you uncomfortable.*

A60: A clinical experience question with a twist. Most of the questions in this section have focused on the positive. But this one pointblank wants you to describe a negative situation. As with all negative questions, you should describe the situation briefly and quickly move on to positives, such as what you learned from the incident. Be realistic; doctors are not perfect. I am sure you have seen a physician make a less than kind joke about a patient, family member, or nurse; witnessed the rude behavior of a patient; or been present when a mistake was made. Speak frankly and show you understand uncomfortable situations happen.

Q61: *Describe a time when you were a patient and received medical care. What did you learn from the experience?*

A61: We've all been a patient at some point in our lives, even if just for preventative care trips to the pediatrician, internist, or family physician. This question provides another chance for you to describe your understanding of medicine, but this time from the patient perspective. If you have experienced a significant illness, this is the time to describe what was likely a profound journey for you and affected your desire to be a physician.

One of the most common questions I am asked regarding medical school admissions is if it will "hurt" an applicant to bring up a medical issue. Many pre-meds fear that describing illness will make them look weak and unfit to be a physician. I have a strong opinion on this one – you should feel comfortable being honest about your experiences. How dare a medical school admissions committee judge you undesirably because you have been what nearly all humans will be at some point in their lives – a patient! Yes, you shouldn't dwell on the negative or tell a 10-minute sob story. Yes, medical schools want healthy students given medicine is both physically and emotionally challenging. And, yes, you should emphasize your current good health and how you know you can handle the academic, physical, and emotional rigor of medicine. But you should not be embarrassed about your patient experiences. I include psychological disease in my definition of "medical" issues. By way of example, the lifetime prevalence of major depression of adults in the US is upwards of 25%. It is a common and treatable condition with likely strong genetic links, just like high blood pressure. Would you be afraid of discussing your high blood pressure in a medical school interview? I'd hope not. There is no need to cover up issues with mental health, especially if you feel they have been formative and worth discussing. The key to presenting personal medical challenges is to be forthright, succinct, and confident with a positive tone.

Clinical experience should be such a foundational part of your desire to be a physician that I hope answering Chapter 12 questions will be relatively easy for you. I suggest you take time now to brainstorm and practice.

CHAPTER 13

Category VIII: Application-related

In this chapter, we will discuss the questions that cause many pre-meds great anxiety because they either focus on the negative aspects of the application or bring up confrontational topics. By the end of this chapter, you will have a strong foundation for answering these queries and no need to fear them.

Q62: *Explain your poor grades [insert semester/year here].*

A62: Almost all pre-meds have some less-than-perfect grades. Be ready to answer questions about why you faltered academically during such periods, stating the negative quickly, and then moving on to the positive (how you improved, what you learned). Stay away from answers implying you partied too much or were bored. More acceptable answers include difficult transition to new environment, working on new study style, over-commitment to non-academic activities, challenging yourself with high-level courses, specific life experience (illness, family situation) making it difficult to focus, *etc.* With these challenging, often negative-leaning questions, it is best to keep the answer short. Why dwell on the negative?

Q63: What happened on the MCAT?

A63: This question implies you did poorly on the MCAT and will likely only be given to applicants with MCAT2015 scores of less than 510 or an uneven score. Most pre-meds get very nervous when asked this question and talk anxiously in circles about what went wrong. I suggest simply stating your performance was not as you hoped, as you had been scoring significantly higher on practice tests (assuming this is true). Then smile, indicating, "Next question please." If you have retaken the MCAT and improved your score, highlight this positive. Also indicate if you are scheduled to take the MCAT again in the future, though the benefits and risks of sitting the exam late in the admissions cycle would be worth a discussion with your pre-med tutor and/or an admissions consultant.

Q64: *There seems to be a mismatch between your GPA and MCAT. Please explain.*

A64: Many pre-meds suffer from a mismatch between GPA and MCAT – either a high GPA and low MCAT or vice versa. Take the same tactic as you have with most negative questions. Provide a brief answer ending on a positive note and move on. End with something like, "As you can see from my strong GPA (or MCAT), I am confident I can handle the academic rigor of medical school."

Q65: *Do you think the MCAT is a good measure or determining factor for admission to medical school?*

A65: Now this is a leading question. The MCAT is controversial, and there is no right answer to this question. Answer honestly. If you respond in the negative, be sure you don't sound like a whiny pre-med. Instead, discuss how many admissions committees are moving towards a more holistic admissions process or that it takes more than book smarts to be a great physician.

Q66: *Tell me about the institutional action against you. How have you changed since then?*

A66: Institutional action can sink an otherwise exceptional medical school applicant. If you have answered, "Yes" to the institutional action questions on the AMCAS, TMDSAS, or AACOMAS applications, you will almost certainly be asked more about it. Have a standard response prepared, following the strategy already outlined for all negative questions. Briefly describe what happened, and then move on to what you learned from it or how you have changed. Do not blame anyone but yourself and avoid sob stories.

Q67: *If you could go back and improve one area of your application, what would it be and why?*

A67: This question feels similar to the "challenge" or "mistake" questions you will become familiar with in Chapter 20. Fortunately, you already have a strategy in place, as this falls into the category of negative questions. Pick an area of your application where you have already improved. This way, you can turn a negative to a positive. Academics are a common answer to this question. You might say, "I wish I could go back and improve my first semester sophomore year academic performance. Fortunately, I worked out the kinks in my study techniques and solved the issues, as seen in the rest of my grades." Or you could go down the extracurricular path: "I wish I had become involved in research sooner in college. Now that I have seen the direct impact of clinical research by working with Dr. Joshi for the past two semesters, I know I could have made a greater difference in the lives of patients.

Fortunately, I can continue with similar research in medical school." Perhaps we should create a mantra, "Briefly state the negative and quickly move on to the positive." It works every time.

Q68: *As a re-applicant, how have you improved your application?*

A68: If you are a re-applicant, you have hopefully already discussed your application with your school's pre-med advisor and/or a professional admissions consultant and clearly remember what areas required improvement. Use these areas as a guide in answering this question. The rule of three works well here, "I have worked to improve three main parts of my application..." Then detail the improvement using specifics.

Q69: *If you are not accepted into medical school this year, what will you do?*

A69: I suggest answering this question by discussing how you will spend the next year gaining experience to improve your application prior to re-applying. Think of this query as a chance to show the interviewer you understand the potential weaknesses of your application. For example,

> "Of course, I hope to be successful this cycle and believe I have the credentials to gain acceptance to medical school. But if it doesn't work out, I will take my clinical research experience abroad to work on HIV medicine implementation studies in Eritrea for six months. Upon returning to the US, I will gain more clinical experience through hospital volunteering and would love to take a medical Spanish course to improve my language skills prior to applying again next June. I won't let the setback of not gaining acceptance this year prevent me from fulfilling my calling to be a physician."

Q70: *What other schools have you applied to?*

A70: Many pre-meds think this question is out of line. Thousands of words fill SDN forums lamenting the horrible admissions interviewers who dare ask such questions. Forget the forums and prepare an answer. My suggestion is to keep it broad, "I have applied to about approximately 20 schools, with a focus on top-tier institutions on both coasts." Or, "I have applied to about 15 schools, focusing on medical schools with strong research traditions." Or maybe, "I have cast a wide net, applying to all of my state schools and many private institutions throughout the Midwest and East Coast." You do not need to name each school. If pushed to give a few specific names, choose three representing the main types of schools where you have applied.

Q71: *Where else have you interviewed?*

A71: Another question causing great angst on SDN forums. If you've already had five interviews, then simply list them. If you haven't had any others, say something like, "You are my first interview, but I have three others lined up this month, including..." or "You are my first interview, and I expect to hear from [insert two or three school names] shortly." Don't let these direct questions ruffle you. The manner in which you answer these questions is often as important as the content of your answers.

We've come to the end of Chapter 13, and it's time for more brainstorming and practice. Remember, brief direct answers without a hint of unease are the keys to most application-oriented queries.

CHAPTER 14

Category IX: Future

Many admissions interviewers have an interest in how you envision your future career. Don't worry, no interviewer will follow up ten years from now and give you a hard time if you didn't stick to the exact path laid out in an interview. I was 100% sure I wanted to be an orthopedic surgeon. After my orthopedic rotation, I knew it wasn't for me and became an emergency physician instead. When asked a "future" question, give your best guess at this time in your career (which is very, very early).

Q72: *Where do you see yourself in 10 years?*

A72: Given medical school generally takes four years, residency three to seven years, and a fellowship a year or two on top of that, you will likely still be in training or at the beginning of your attending status in 10 years. You may answer this question by discussing your understanding of the medical training schedule, providing specifics about specialties you are considering, and expressing interest in practice locations (urban vs. rural, academic vs. community, hospital vs. private practice). You might also impress an interviewer by bringing up future goals other than those regarding your specialty choice, such as continued research, education, policy work, international health, another degree, *etc*. Finally, it's nice to work in your personal interests, such as goals for family life and free time.

As with all questions, honesty is the best policy when answering these future-oriented questions. For example, even though the US is in need of more primary care physicians and many medical schools find an interest in primary care a bonus with regards to admissions, do not state an interest in primary care unless it is true and can be substantiated through your prior experience. Stating your goals honestly and with passion will serve you better than trying to guess what your interviewer wants to here.

Q73: *What specialty are you considering?*

A73: You have already prepared this answer based on your Q72 response. Doesn't that feel great?

Q74: *In 25 years, looking back on your medical career, how will you determine if you have been successful?*

A74: This question is not asking you to predict your specialty. It's asking about your definition of professional success. You can employ the rule of three here if you wish, discussing the three main areas in which you want to be judged, such as clinical practice, research, and teaching. Or you can take a more specific approach and describe exactly what you think a successful career looks like.

Q75: *If you were to change one thing about the future what would it be?*

A75: There are a million possible answers to this question, and your response might have nothing to do with medicine. This is another opportunity to show you are well-rounded and have a diversity of interests. When brainstorming possible answers, think about topics you can discuss in depth, because you are very likely to trigger further conversation with whatever response you choose. I have heard excellent answers to this question on topics ranging from removing national borders to making toll roads illegal to creating a universal language to destroying all weapons. Have fun with this one.

That's it for the Chapter 14 future questions. During your brainstorm and practice time, enjoy thinking of what your future will bring and dream big!

CHAPTER 15

Category X: Diversity

If you have filled out medical school secondary applications, I am sure you have come across many versions of "diversity" questions. Similar questions come up frequently in medical school interviews because admissions committees are tasked with creating diverse classes.

Q76: *What does diversity mean to you?*

A76: This question opens the door for you to broadly define diversity. Pre-meds often think of diversity only along race or ethnicity lines. But there is so much more to it: diversity of age, gender, sexual orientation, religion, nationality, upbringing, education, and, most importantly, life experience. When defining what diversity means to you, think broadly. Also consider how you add to the diversity of a medical school class.

Q77: *How will you add to the diversity of this school?*

A77: You have likely already answered this question in secondary essays, and you may feel free to provide a similar answer in interviews. The rule of three also works very well here. As mentioned in the previous question discussion, diversity can be broadly defined. Here are some responses I have heard from pre-meds who successfully gained admissions to medical school. Use the list to help you brainstorm.

- Collegiate athlete who brings unique mixture of self-motivation, teamwork, and leadership
- President of global health club with deep passion for cultural competence in medicine
- Small-business owner who brings entrepreneurship and business knowledge
- Non-traditional student who will augment diversity through five years of experience in "real world" working in IT
- Survivor of a car accident with multiple injuries who will add a deep understanding of what it is like to be a patient
- Speaker of three languages who has lived abroad and brings first-hand multi-cultural perspective
- Career-changing attorney with well-honed analytic and leadership skills easily transferrable to medicine
- Devout Muslim from small town in the Midwest who has overcome racism on a daily basis
- Resident assistant in charge of dozens of other students who brings strong listening and relationship skills
- Passionate hiker who has completed the Appalachian Trail and will add perseverance, wilderness EMT skills, and an independent streak
- Daughter who lost mom to cancer who brings understanding of how to care for others in the their moments of greatest need
- Founder of non-profit focused on decreasing poverty of Indian farmers who will add managerial and international knowledge to the class

- Man who recently came out as gay who will add the importance of being true to oneself while being non-judgmental and tolerant of others
- Self-taught musician who will help develop a culture of creativity
- Future primary care physician who has volunteered in a rural clinic for three summers and will remind fellow students of the medical service gaps in our own country
- Son of divorced parents who has volunteered with children in similar situations and brings compassion for those who have felt abandoned
- Craft blogger with 5,000 followers who will add strong writing and communication skills, along with a passion for creating with one's hands
- Artist who paints for charity and will bring a passion for philanthropy and the healing qualities of art
- Child of immigrants who worked two jobs to pay for college and adds skills of hard work, humility, and time management
- Computer programmer who created wellness app and will bring ability to combine medicine and technology to promote health change

Q78: *Describe a time you were in a minority.*

A78: Many pre-meds immediately focus on race or ethnicity when the word minority is used. But as with diversity, minority can have a broad meaning. Perhaps you were the only American on a trip abroad, the only male participating in a stereotypically female task, or the only non-science major in a certain class. You should not answer this question with, "I've never been a minority." We've all been a minority of some sort. In addition to describing the situation, I also suggest you weave in how it made you feel and what you learned from it.

Q79: *What values do you bring from your cultural background that will be useful in medicine?*

A79: Since everyone has a cultural background, everyone can answer this question. Even if you are a sixth-generation American or don't think of yourself as coming from a particularly interesting culture, you still have a background filled with values that will be useful in medicine. Review the list of characteristics medical schools are looking for in applicants from Chapter 1. Reading the qualities list will remind you of the values you might discuss in your response. Oh, and remember the rule of three I've been hitting you over the head with? It works well here. Of course, you don't want to answer every interview question with a three-part answer. But since it is such a natural way to answer a question, you can certainly use the rule of three multiple times in the same interview session.

Q80: *At [insert school name here], we work with underserved populations such as Hispanics and African Americans. Have you had experience with underserved populations?*

A80: Hopefully you have had some experience with underserved populations and can pull from those experiences to answer this question. If you have not, consider gaining some experience with the disadvantaged before heading to medical school, as these populations are often the ones you will be serving the most as a medical student and physician-in-training. Though it is ideal if the experience is clinical, you may serve others in many ways, such as tutoring, helping the homeless, being a big buddy, *etc.*

Many pre-meds have told me answering diversity questions can at times feel disingenuous. I think that's because individuals who are not from underrepresented minority backgrounds take too narrow a view of diversity, as I've mentioned above. When you brainstorm Chapter 15's questions, try to find moments to discuss that feel authentic. You are certainly unique, so show it!

CHAPTER 16

Category XI: Coping Skills

You know medicine is a challenging profession. You've likely heard physicians complain about work hours and administrative burdens during shadowing experiences, listened to negative newscasts about Obamacare, and read articles on our "broken" healthcare system. Given the well-known difficulties of the field you wish to enter, medical school interviewers often want to know how you cope with challenges.

Q81: *Medicine is a depressing business - how will you cope?*

A81: We all have coping skills to deal with emotionally-charged situations. Whether it's exercise, talking with friends and family, focusing on the positive, having a cathartic cry then moving on, reading novels, participating in religious traditions, or using many of the other possible coping mechanisms, you need to describe how you deal with emotional stress. It is common for pre-meds to provide a general answer to this question and forget to describe specific coping strategies. Remember to provide details.

Q82: *How will you handle the stress of medical school?*

A82: You can easily adapt your answer to Q81 to answer this query, even though it focuses more on general stress than emotional stress. If you have suffered from physical or mental illness, this is a another good time to confidently provide evidence that you have the ability to complete the demands of medical school and excel as a physician in a physically- and emotionally-demanding field.

Q83: *What do you do to blow off steam?*

A83: Again, you can adapt your response to Q81 and Q82 to create the answer to this query.

Q84: *How do you know you will enjoy taking care of sick people?*

A84: This question involves part clinical experience and part coping skills. Your answer may begin with a response created for the clinical experience set of questions, proving you know what it's like to care for the ill and injured, and then finish with a coping skills description.

Q85: *Have you ever seen someone die? How did you handle this?*

A85: If you have seen someone die, begin your answer with a brief description of the circumstances and end with specifics of how you coped with this particular incident. If you have never seen anyone die, answer, "No," and then discuss a time you saw someone very sick or close to death. If you have never seen someone who is very ill, many doctors and members of medical school admissions committees would argue you should gain more clinical experience. Handling the emotional stress of severe illness is a key skill for any physician.

Q86: *How would you handle being unable to help someone or making a serious clinical mistake?*

A86: This query is really two questions. You may either answer each question separately or choose which you want to answer, given the word "or" implies choice. The best way to answer either question is with a specific example of a time when you or someone you observed could not help someone or made a serious mistake (of course moving on to the positives of what you learned from it as soon as possible). If you don't have a specific experience to draw from, then discuss your general coping skills prepared for Q81 to Q85.

Q87: *How will you deal with leaving your family and moving to a new location?*

A87: This question asks for a very specific set of coping skills, namely those required when moving to a new place. I suggest focusing your answer on the tactics you employ when trying to settle into a new environment, make new friends, or find a new community. This provides an excellent opportunity to discuss the ways you enjoy spending time outside the classroom.

Q88: *Have you ever been overwhelmed? How did you handle this?*

A88: "No" is not an appropriate answer to this question. We have all been overwhelmed. You could use the example created from the "how would you handle being unable to help someone...?" part of Q86 or devise a novel response. How you handled being overwhelmed is the most important part of the question. Feeling overwhelmed academically is the most common response, but try to be more creative than describing the usual pre-med academic stresses. This question offers another opportunity for you to show well-roundedness and discuss parts of your life that might not have made it on the application.

We've come to the end of Chapter 16. You know what to do – brainstorm and practice!

CHAPTER 17

Category XII: Professionalism/ Physician Role

Professionalism is a hot topic in medical school admissions. Questions about professionalism and the physician's role in society likely appeared on some of your secondary applications. Doctors take their exalted place in society seriously and want to ensure pre-meds understand the virtues of the club they are trying to enter.

Q89: Define professionalism.

A89: I will admit this is a painful question, but it often comes up in medical school interviews. It's hard to know where to begin with such queries, but you already have a head start. The list of characteristics in Chapter 1 is filled with adjectives to help you define professionalism. I would employ the rule of three here and start with something like, "I believe professionalism can be defined by three main qualities..." Name the qualities and give examples showing how the qualities directly relate to professionalism. These examples can be from your life or hypothetical.

Q90: *Describe the ideal physician.*

A90: Dare I mention the characteristics list again? Think about the doctor you look up to the most. What qualities does he or she possess? Envision him or her as you create your answer. You can even mention this physician in your response, if you wish. It adds a nice personal touch and allows you to reiterate your clinical experience.

Q91: *What is the role of physicians in society?*

A91: You may take this answer anywhere you like. Physicians have many societal roles, from healers to leaders to educators. You may give your opinion about a doctor's main role in society or discuss their many roles. Again you might use a specific physician you know or describe a hypothetical one.

Q92: *Tell me about a time when a physician acted inappropriately. How did you react?*

A92: Though it may be hard for you to talk negatively about a physician, this question is forcing you to do so. Doctors are not perfect, and even your ideal physician has made and will continue to make mistakes. Remember the "tell me about an experience during your shadowing that made you uncomfortable" question (Q60) from Chapter 12? You could adapt that answer here, if what made you uncomfortable was related to a physician acting inappropriately. If you can't adapt that answer, you will have to brainstorm another situation. To help get you started, here are some areas where physicians could act inappropriately: communicating with patients, family, or other staff; reacting to a medical error; breaking a rule or policy; making fraudulent insurance claims; setting a bad example for patients; using humor inappropriately; or abusing substances.

Q93: Name a time when you saw someone acting unprofessionally. What did you do and why?

A93: You may use either the answer prepared for Q92 or branch out into other areas of your life. Remember to answer the "why" part of the question, as it is easy to forget the second query in multi-part questions.

Q94: In an operating room, there's the surgeon, anesthesiologist, nurses, technicians, etc. Who is the most important person in that room?

A94: It's only natural to begin your answer with, "They are all equally important." But be prepared for interviewers who will push you on this answer and force you to state which role is "most" important. There is no right answer, and it is not a given that you should answer, "The surgeon is the most important." Whomever you choose, you must back up your choice with a persuasive argument. One way to approach this question is to describe the responsibilities of each person mentioned, and then reveal who you think is most important based on your descriptions. You might also consider a person in the room not mentioned in the question: the patient!

Q95: If a doctor is the coach of a sport, what sport do you think best fits and why?

A95: Though wrapped up in a fun disguise, this question is really asking what many of the professionalism questions are asking – how would you describe a physician's professional role. By picking a sport, you are providing a segway to the characteristics you think excellent physicians should possess. If I had to answer this question, I'd choose basketball, because doctors excel in fast-paced, team-oriented environments filled with hundreds of decisions and often nail-biting outcomes.

That's it for Chapter 17 questions and for Week 3, which covered many secondary-like topics and some direct questions targeting potential application weaknesses. Brainstorm and practice professionalism and physician role questions today, and then review the entire week tomorrow.

WEEK 4

Week 4 includes more questions that will feel similar to secondary application prompts and some challenging queries asking you to describe your soft skills, sell yourself, and think outside the box. It is normal for this week to feel more difficult than the previous three weeks. However, the daily routine of reading a chapter, brainstorming answers to each question presented, and answering each question out loud (hopefully recorded on video and reviewed) should start to feel like second nature.

Day 1
Read Chapter 18 (Category XIII: Characteristics)
Brainstorm answers to questions
Practice answering each question out loud

Day 2
Read Chapter 19 (Category XIV: Soft Skills/Inner Self)
Brainstorm answers to questions
Practice answering each question out loud

Day 3
Read Chapter 20 (Category XV: Challenge)
Brainstorm answers to questions
Practice answering each question out loud

Day 4
Read Chapter 21 (Category XVI: School Specific)

Brainstorm answers to questions

Practice answering each question out loud

Day 5

Read Chapter 22 (Category XVII: Sell Yourself)

Brainstorm answers to questions

Practice answering each question out loud

Day 6

Read Chapter 23 (Category XVIII: Outside the Box)

Brainstorm answers to questions

Practice answering each question out loud

Day 7

Review Chapters 18-23

Practice any questions you found challenging

CHAPTER 18

Category XIII: Characteristics

Characteristics have come up often in our discussion of medical school interview preparation. Many interviewers, in an attempt to get to know you more deeply than through what is written on your application pages, will probe your personality with characteristics questions. If not prepared, many pre-meds struggle with these. But once you know what questions could come your way, answering queries about your qualities becomes quite easy (with practice, of course).

Q96: *What are your strengths?*

A96: Many pre-meds worry about sounding arrogant when answering this question. The question is asking you to toot your own horn, so don't worry about sounding vain. Pick three strengths you can support with evidence from your own life. For example,

> "I excel as a leader. As elected co-captain of my college's soccer team, I have learned the power of motivating others and take great pride in our turn from an initially losing season into a championship run. I am also proud of my time-management skills, which have allowed me to balance academics, college

sports, tutoring children with autism, and volunteering at the local free clinic. Finally, I think I am good listener. Friends often turn to me in times of stress, and I gain great satisfaction helping them find solutions to their problems."

Choose three strengths that show your multi-faceted personality, such as compassion, resilience, and analytical skills, instead of picking three similar characteristics, such as compassion, empathy, and kindness. This question offers another opportunity to show you are well-rounded.

Q97: *What are your weaknesses?*

A97: Given the question asks for weaknesses (plural) you have to give more than one. But as you don't want to harp on the negative, I suggest breaking the rule of three here and providing two weaknesses. Of course, you should state the weaknesses briefly, and then move the answer toward the positive. For example,

"Early in college, I tended to overcommit, saying yes to every opportunity offered. But when I realized I provided a disservice to my peers by trying to do everything instead of focusing my energy on a few important tasks, I learned how to politely say no and immediately saw an improvement in my ability to succeed. Whether with my dance troupe, pre-med club, or research laboratory, I have continued focusing my time on performing fewer tasks at a higher level. I also tend to be quite sensitive. While this helps me with empathy, it sometimes leads me to avoid confrontation, even when speaking my mind could be helpful. I have worked to develop a thicker skin and found dealing with challenging situations early often prevents hard feelings in the future."

Even though this answer provides two negatives, it actually makes the responder appear mature, introspective, and willing to work on his faults.

Q98: *Name some good qualities you possess and one quality you'd like to work on or change.*

A98: You may use the strengths from Q96 and a weakness from Q97 to answer this query.

Q99: *Name five words off the top of your head that describe you.*

A99: This question often stumps pre-meds with most initially responding with a long, "Ummmmm." You already have three words to describe yourself prepared (your strengths from Q96). I suggest adding a fourth strength and throwing in a weakness to show you are human. Again, pick diverse strengths to highlight your multi-faceted personality.

Q100: *How would your friends describe you?*

A100: I propose using the same answer you have prepared for Q98. Provide three strengths and one weakness.

Q101: *How would your brother/sister/cousin describe you?*

A101: Even though this question is trying to be tricky by bringing your family into the mix, it is asking the same thing as most of the questions in this chapter, *i.e.*, what are your strengths and weaknesses? Fortunately, you already have an answer prepared that can be easily tweaked to respond to this specific query.

Q102: *Think about people who don't like you. What would they say about you?*

A102: Most people who don't like you would talk about your weaknesses. Answer this question by providing a weakness or two.

Q103: *Think about the people you don't like. What don't you like about them?*

A103: Finally, a question not directly about you. But your response does reflect on how you perceive the world. Giving three negative characteristics about those you don't like says as much about you as your own strengths and weaknesses. I'd answer by saying, "I don't like people who are selfish, arrogant, or lazy."

Hopefully you have found Chapter 18 to be relatively straightforward given what you've already learned in this book. Brainstorm and practice the characteristics questions and get ready for a challenging Chapter 19.

Category XIV: Soft Skills/ Inner Self

With medical school admissions shifting focus from academics alone and to a more holistic approach, many interviewers will try to evaluate your soft skills through a variety of challenging questions. I find these to be some of the hardest queries to answer. But, as with anything, knowing what to expect and practicing will enable you to smoothly respond to even the most difficult questions that come your way.

Q104: *Provide me with an example of your leadership ability.*

A104: This is an easy one. Physicians, by default, are leaders of the medical team. Thus, interviewers want to assess your leadership skills. If you don't have an obvious answer, such as serving as an elected member of a club, a captain of an athletic team, or the founder of a school activity, then draw on less formal experiences, such as leading a friend out of a troubling situation, unofficially mentoring others, or planning a valuable experience.

Q105: *What does being a leader mean to you?*

A105: These types of questions often lead to generic, preachy, or cheesy answers. Avoid these traps by providing the characteristics of a leader, and then give examples of leaders you have seen exhibit these characteristics. By providing specific examples, you will create an interesting answer and avoid the generic/preachy/cheesy traps. If you don't want to go the qualities route, you may describe a life experience with leadership, either when you or another has been a successful leader, and finish off the description with what the experience meant to you.

Q106: *How do you manage your time?*

A106: Time management is a big topic in medicine as physicians are often pulled in many directions at once. There is no trick to answering this question. Similar to the coping queries in Chapter 16, the interviewers want to hear your strategy when faced with multi-tasking and time limitations. I suggest picking at specific period in your life where time management was a challenge and discuss how you successfully managed your time. The use of these details will make the answer more memorable compared to answering with a description of your generic time management skills.

Q107: *Rate your humbleness on a scale of 1-10.*

A107: Now that is a catch-22. Rating your humility highly is, by definition, not humble. Rating it on the lower side of the scale makes you look arrogant. I suggest picking somewhere in the middle and backing up your answer with evidence from your life. Or, if you'd like to throw the curve ball back at the interviewer, you could discuss the catch-22, and then settle on the median 5! Just make sure you do this with a smile on your face.

Q108: *What's the difference between talent and skill?*

A108: Yikes. Are these questions getting harder? I warned you these "soft skills" questions can be a challenge. An obvious way to prepare for this question is to look up the definitions in a dictionary. But the exact word definitions are less important than what the words mean to you. There is no right answer. For example, "I view a talent as innate, something you are born with that can be nurtured. A skill, on the other hand, I see as an expertise that can be learned and not necessarily requiring a natural inclination." By using phrases such as, "I view" and, "I see," you are intimating these are your opinions, and you are not presenting the definitions as facts.

Q109: *Define success.*

A109: Take your answer to this question anywhere you wish. You may talk about success professionally, personally, specifically, or generally. Do you remember this question?: "In 25 years, looking back on your medical career, how will you determine if you have been successful?" (Q74 in Chapter 14). Refer to your response to this question as fodder for answering, "Define success." But don't feel like you have to speak only about medicine. Success may have a much broader meaning for you. And you now know how much medical school admissions committees like well-rounded pre-meds!

Q110: *Define empathy and give an example.*

A110: Instead of looking up the definition of empathy, try to define it yourself now. Once you have come up with a definition, see how closely it comes to the official dictionary definition. I bet it is pretty close. As you have likely noticed, medical school interviewers seem to enjoy asking you to define characteristics required in doctors. You aren't going to be able to memorize the definition of every such characteristic, and this would be a waste of time. Instead, go through the list of characteristics in Chapter 1 and devise a definition off the top of your head for each. Then turn to the dictionary. If your definition of any term is markedly different than the dictionary, then it's worth learning the official meaning. Otherwise, keep your own definition and tie it to a personal example. This way, you will be able to quickly devise your own definition during an interview, which is much easier than attempting to think of a memorized dictionary definition.

Q111: *Define maturity.*

A111: Use the same technique as for Q110. And even though the query does not ask you to give an example, you now understand the power of tying responses to personal experiences. So go ahead and give an example from your own life anyway.

Q112: *What are you most proud of that is not on your resume?*

A112: I love this question. Since most of your academic, research, community service, extracurricular, and clinical experiences are on your resume, you will have to think outside the box to devise an answer. Many pre-meds have successfully answered this question by drawing moments from personal relationships, life challenges, or times when they took a risk and it paid off. Don't think too hard about this one. Going with what pops into your mind often works best because it is heartfelt. Some great answers I have heard involve overcoming a fear of heights to zip line through the forest, reading to a son every night, making the high school basketball team on the fourth try, turning down a dream trip abroad to stay home and care for an ailing grandmother, and completing a 10K race after six months of training when the longest previous run was 1 mile.

Q113: *What has been your most defining moment?*

A113: When brainstorming your defining moment, consider your strengths we have discussed in Chapter 18. Now think of a moment in your life that shows you have most or all of these qualities. I suggest that is your defining moment.

Q114: *Name one situation that impacted you the most.*

A114: You can modify your answers to Q112 or Q113 for a response to this question. No need to reinvent the wheel, especially with such difficult queries. And do note it is unlikely you will be asked multiple questions on the same topic in an interview. For example, most interviewers will not ask you to describe both your defining moment and a situation that has impacted you the most. Thus, you are usually safe preparing a similar answer to both questions.

Q115: *What is your passion?*

A115: If you have one obvious overarching passion, describe it in your answer. However, most of us don't have just one. You may consider discussing a passion in various areas, such as academics, clinical experience, and hobbies, to show the broad scope of your interests.

Q116: *What do you love?*

A116: If you have ever watched *Inside the Actors Studio* with James Lipton, this next series of questions may make you giggle. Despite their similarity to what Lipton asks his famous guests, these questions all come directly from real medical school interviews. Just as Lipton wants to probe the inner depths of actors, medical school interviewers hope to grab a glimpse of the "real" you through such queries. I think the best way to answer these types of questions is with your gut. What first pops into your head when someone asks, "What do you love?" "My puppy Alexander, warm chocolate chip cookies right out of the oven, and the feeling I get when I cross the finish line at the Boston Marathon" is an example of an honest, interesting, and perfectly acceptable answer. Don't be afraid to let your guard down a bit and share something of yourself interviewers can't find on your application.

Q117: *What drives you?*

A117: It is more powerful to answer this question with a specific description: "I am driven by the happiness and relief I have seen on the faces of the patients I help at the local clinic, such as Anna, who has recently been cured of breast cancer," as opposed to the more abstract: "I am driven by feeling the satisfaction that comes from helping others on a daily basis." The difference between these two possible responses highlights why I so often suggest pulling answers from your specific life experiences. As you know by now, your answer doesn't have to be medically related.

Q118: *What makes you laugh?*

A118: Think of yourself laughing and what triggered the feeling of humor. If the topic is appropriate for a medical school interview (*i.e.*, not vulgar or potty humor), then you have your answer. Avoid telling a joke that could be taken the wrong way.

Q119: *What makes you angry?*

A119: Think of yourself enraged and the trigger for the feeling of anger. Again, if the topic is appropriate, you have your answer.

Q120: *What do you find frustrating?*

A120: Use the same strategy as Q118 and Q119.

Q121: *Do you have any biases?*

A121: We all have biases, so you will have to answer, "Yes" or, "Of course." But it is your explanation of the bias that is important. As biases are typically negative, you will once again want to quickly turn the negative into a positive. Here's an example of how I'd answer this question,

> "I have struggled in the past with feelings of frustration toward able-bodied people who refuse to work and take welfare. Of course, I have to remind myself, 'Who am I to judge?' It is likely I am not privy to many of the reasons individuals lean on the welfare system."

Q122: *Would you rather be a compassionate or a competent physician?*

A122: I hope you will be both compassionate and competent, but in asking this question, the interviewer wants you to choose and provide support for your beliefs. Where do you find support? From your own life experiences, of course! Think about the doctors you admire. Do you think they are more compassionate or more competent? Use the answer to this question to respond to Q122.

Did this chapter feel tiring? If so, that is only natural. Some pre-meds have told me these soft skills/inner self queries feel like a therapy session. The questions certainly aren't traditional and often take us out of our comfort zone. Spend the rest of today brainstorming and practicing Chapter 19's questions. And if you found this chapter particularly challenging, then run through it at least twice.

CHAPTER 20

Category XV: Challenge

Challenge or mistake questions epitomize the negative question. But you already know how to deal with such queries, right? Directly and succinctly state the negative and quickly move on to the positive (*i.e.*, what you learned from the challenge or mistake). You will likely already have considered some of these challenge questions in your secondary prompts and may use the same themes to answer interview challenge queries.

There are many ways medical school admissions interviewers try to push you to reveal your weaknesses. They are not asking such negative questions to prove you are human; they are asking to see how you respond to hardship. It is often in negative moments that our true selves are defined.

Q123: *What is the biggest mistake you have ever made, and what did you learn from it?*

A123: The trick in this question is to be honest without making yourself appear to be a horrible person. Refrain from speaking about academic dishonesty or breaking the law. Instead, think about personal conflicts, missed opportunities, or poor judgments, as these kind of topics often lend themselves to a positive discussion of lessons learned. Here are three possible answers:

1. "During my junior year in college, my sister and I had a terrible falling out. I responded by avoiding the issue and did not communicate with her for over six months. After hours of reflection and seeking the advice of family and friends, I reached out to her and was able to mend the relationship. Being the first to break the silence was one of the hardest things I have ever done given the depth of hurt she had caused me, but it taught me the power of humility and opening oneself to emotional risk. Though our relationship is far from perfect, we both now realize the importance of being present in each others' lives."

2. "Two summers ago, I was given the opportunity to travel to India on a two-month surgical mission. Given the cost, I turned down the offer and regretted it for months. International health is my passion, and I promised to never let money stand in the way of following my desire to help those most in need. I found another opportunity, this time in Burma, and fundraised over $5000 in order to make the trip happen. I just returned and can confidently say the trip was a life-changing experience that confirmed my decision to become a doctor."

3. "When I was 20, I tore my ACL while playing basketball with friends. After surgery and intense rehabilitation, I was instructed to avoid any sports requiring a quick change of direction for six months. Ignoring my doctor's advice, I went skiing with friends and tore the ACL again, requiring further surgery and over a year of rehab. In addition to learning I am not super human, I also realized the importance of trusting experts. This experience will certainly help me better communicate with my patients in

the future as an orthopedic surgeon, because I understand the motivations that may lead them to disregard best advice."

Q124: *Do you feel you have had to overcome any hardships/struggles?*

A124: Your "mistake" answer may or may not adequately answer this question. The first example answer for Q123 could work here, but the second and third don't quite fit because a mistake is not necessarily a hardship or struggle. If your mistake answer works for this query, go ahead and use it. If not, think about a time in your life when you had to fight for something, felt you were barely keeping your head above water, or persevered despite obstacles. Brainstorming about such experiences should trigger an answer to the hardships/struggles question.

Q125: *What are you most ashamed of?*

A125: Again, your mistake answer may work here or it may not. The first and third examples from Q123 could both be tweaked to respond to a question about shame. If your mistake answer doesn't quite fit, ponder times when your cheeks burned in embarrassment, you couldn't get a certain action out of your mind because you behaved badly, or you wanted to run away from something. These are the feelings that often come with shame. Of course, remember to choose an answer that will end on a positive note.

Q126: *What is your biggest regret in life?*

A126: The second and third example from Q123 could be used here because missed opportunities and poor choices often lead to regret. Personal conflict, neglect of personal life, money misuse, loss of an opportunity, or time mismanagement are all fodder for regret question responses.

Q127:   *Describe a time in which you failed at something in a non-academic setting.*

A127:   Failure is in the eye of the beholder. It can be defined in many ways: lack of success, the omission of a required action, defeat, disaster, inadequacy, deficiency, shortfall, negligence, oversight, *etc.* Failure can involve only yourself or others. You can fail through action or inaction. And failure is not necessarily bad, as the most intense learning often comes from failure. As we have all experienced many failures, I suggest choosing one for your response which led to success or served as a great learning experience.

Q128:   *What was a time you made a poor choice?*

A128:   The third example answer from Q123 would work perfectly here, as could the many possible responses to Q127. Review your answers to all of the previous questions, and I bet you will find a poor choice was involved in one of them.

Q129:   *Describe a time when you let someone down and how you resolved the situation.*

A129:   We don't always live up to expectations, so this should be an easy question for all of us. Choose a time when you let someone down, realized the mistake, and took action to rectify the situation. If you want to be a bit creative, describe a time when you let yourself down. After all, we are often our own biggest critics.

Q130:   *Describe a personal conflict you've had with somebody and how you dealt with it.*

139

A130: By preparing answers to the previous questions in this chapter, you likely have a response to this one. If not, think about a time you butted heads with family, friends, or colleagues. What caused the tension and how did you resolve the problem?

Q131: *If you could go back and relive one day in your life, what day would that be? Would you change something about it? If so, what?*

A131: The easiest response entails modifying your answer to Q123. You might also discuss a day when a tragedy occurred, or when you were rejected or disappointed. Another approach is to choose to relive a day because it was spectacular. If you take this path, be sure to think out loud and let the interviewer know you are interpreting this answer differently than most. For example, "Although many people would relive a day to change something bad that happened, I'd like to relive a day where everything seemed to go right." Then you can describe that day.

Q132: *Tell me about the lowest point in your life.*

A132: These questions are getting awfully depressing. Fortunately, it is likely you will receive only one or two negative questions per interview. For this query, you can use either your biggest mistake answer or choose another time you felt down, discouraged, or helpless. Remember to explain how the low point led to a positive experience.

Q133: *What is the worst thing that has ever happened to you?*

A133: Consider two ways to interpret this question. First, you caused the worst thing to happen, or second, another force caused the worst thing to happen. Facing a challenge or making a mistake might not necessarily be the worst thing that has ever happened to you, so think broadly on this one.

Q134: *How do you work with a teammate who is not pulling his or her weight?*

A134: It's easy to immediately think about sports when the word "teammate" is used. Instead, think of a teammate as anyone you have worked with to meet a goal. Though academics is a commonly used subject for this answer, you can, of course, talk about extracurricular experiences. Be sure to use a personal example in your answer. By describing a time you dealt with a teammate not performing up to expectations, you will provide a more memorable answer than by generically discussing how you would theoretically handle the situation. Personal is almost always better than generic in medical school interview answers.

Q135: *Give me an example of a time when you were on a team and it didn't work out? What would you do differently?*

A135: You may use either the response prepared for Q134 or speak about another time your team failed to achieve a goal. This team could involve athletics, arts, business, government, research, academics, *etc.*

Q136: *When were you glad you gave someone a second chance?*

A136: Finally, a question with a positive orientation! Think of a time someone disappointed you and instead of ending the relationship, you gave him or her another opportunity. Relating such experiences is a great way to answer this question.

Q137: *Tell me about a time you felt misjudged by somebody, and how you responded to that situation.*

A137: Of course, only choose an example when you responded well to being misjudged. Discuss any aspect of your life here, from academics to extracurriculars to experiences that did not make it on your application.

Q138: *Describe a time you misjudged someone.*

A138: I am sure you are not surprised by the negative spin from the previous question. Pick a time you made an incorrect judgment and the person proved you wrong. You may also reach back to your answer for "do you have any biases?" (Q121, Chapter 19). Biases often involve misjudgment.

Q139: *Have you ever been discriminated against?*

A139: As discussed in Chapter 15 (Category X: Diversity), discrimination does not always deal with race or ethnicity. Discrimination, unfortunately, takes many forms. Consider modifying your answer to Q137 or using new content. Misjudgment often stems from making split decisions based on discriminatory ideas.

Q140: *When was the last time you felt humbled?*

A140: You should have many possible answers to this question from your mistake, regret, and failure responses.

Q141: *Have you ever harmed anyone?*

A141: Harm does not have to mean physical harm. Hopefully, you have not physically harmed anyone. You can harm others through misjudgment, lack of kindness, exclusion, harsh words, or poor choices. Answering that you have never harmed anyone isn't good enough.

Q142: *Describe a time you needed to ask for help.*

A142: Asking for help is difficult and you will face many times in your career when requesting assistance will be required.

Thus, medical school interviewers want to ensure you know how to ask for help. Though many pre-meds turn to an academic example for their response, I challenge you to move beyond academics. Considering times you needed to ask for help outside the classroom usually leads to a more compelling answer. Look back over your responses to the other challenge questions because you may have asked for help in some of those scenarios.

Q143: *Tell me about a time when you had to assert yourself.*
A143: To answer this query, think about times you had to challenge the norm, stick up for something you believed in, or step out of your comfort zone to succeed.

Q144: *What challenges do you expect to encounter as a physician?*
A144: This should be an easy question to answer, as much of the media attention these days focuses on the many issues facing the US medical system. You can elevate the impressiveness of your answer by relating information you have learned speaking with physicians. In doing so, you will show the interviewer how you have thoroughly explored the medical field and learned both the good and the bad. For example,

"While shadowing Dr. Brown, an internist in private practice, I saw how he faced numerous time pressures when trying to treat patients. He told me he was allowed seven minutes per patient. But what I loved about Dr. Brown was that he spent as much time with each patient as required. Sure, he ran late. But his patients loved him because he made each feel like he or she was the most important patient of the day. In addition, Dr. Brown and I discussed the many systems issues facing doctors today, including insurance glitches, increased administrative burdens, and hyper-specialization. I am eager to learn more about these issues so that I can be part of the solution as a physician."

Once again, presenting a personal experience leads to a strong and memorable answer.

Q145: *What is the hardest question you have ever been asked? How did you answer it?*

A145: Pick one of the many, many difficult questions from this book and give your excellent answer.

We've made it to the end of Chapter 20. Did it feel like a bit of a downer? Don't worry if it did. Once you've brainstormed and practiced the challenge questions, you have a more positive week awaiting you in Chapter 21.

Category XVI: School Specific

Medical schools want to be wanted. It follows that admissions interviewers will ask about your specific desire to attend their institution. Fortunately, you have already had to answer similar questions in many secondary essays. Before you head to any medical school interview, be sure you have a plan for selling the interviewer on why his or her school is perfect for you.

Q146: *Why [insert school name]?*

A146: I think this answer is pretty easy to devise. Think about the three things you are looking for in a medical school. Some examples are: culture of cooperation, problem-based curriculum, world-class faculty, early clinical exposure, research opportunities, service focus, global health experiences, support for extracurriculars, diverse patient population, reputation of affiliated hospitals, residency success rates, and location. Once you have chosen the three, research what the school provides. Be as specific as possible and, using the rule of threes, tell the interviewer where you are going with the answer. For example,

"I want to attend Man's Greatest Medical School for three main reasons. First, I learn best in a problem-based learning curriculum where students cooperate instead of compete. MGMS's innovative curriculum will allow me to learn from both world-class faculty and my fellow students, while also offering early clinical exposure. Second, I hope to become a clinician-scientist in the field of stem cell research. By joining a lab run by great minds, such as Dr. Savant and Dr. Cellborn, I will continue to learn about the cutting edge of research in this area. Finally, I am a Californian born and bred. I'd love to stay near family and friends, my main support network, while attending medical school and preparing myself to best serve Californians as a physician."

Q147: *What are you looking for in a medical school?*

A147: You can easily adapt your answer to Q146 to respond to this query by changing the opening: "I am looking for a medical school with three main characteristics." Then launch into your three.

Q148: *Describe your ideal medical school.*

A148: Too easy! You can again use your "Why [insert school name]?" response with a new lead in to directly answer this question. Isn't it nice to have three questions answered with the preparation of just one?

Q149: *Why not go to your state school where tuition is cheaper?*

A149: Good question. Medical school is expensive, especially private school. You can respond by highlighting what this particular school offers, *i.e.*, use the three characteristics already devised for the previous three answers. Never, never belittle your state school. Negativity will get you nowhere. Focus on the school where you are interviewing and keep it positive.

Q150: *If you were accepted to all the schools where you applied, how would you decide which school to attend?*

A150: Initially, this may seem like a challenging question. But it's really just the "Why [insert specific school]?" question in disguise. You can say something like, "I would make my decision based on various factors, including…" Then give the three (or more if you'd like) characteristics used for the other school specific questions.

Q151: *If you got into Harvard or UCSF, would you come here?*

A151: Don't be shocked by this question. No blushing or jaw dropping. Start with a strong, "Yes," and then give your reasons. As you have already guessed, these will be the reasons prepared for the previous questions.

Q152: *What is your top choice medical school?*

A152: Hmm. This doesn't initially seem to fit the pattern of the previous questions, so I suggest taking a lead from politics on this one. Unless the school where you are interviewing is indeed your top choice, don't give a specific answer. You may side step the question: "Given I am still in the interview process and have more schools to visit, I haven't decided on my top choice. But I will make my final decision based on the most important characteristics and qualities of a medical school for me, such as…" Then sneak in those three characteristics again.

Q153: *If [insert school name] was theoretically your first choice school, what would be your second choice school?*

A153: This is a hard question to side step. Assuming the interviewer inserted his own institution in the [insert school name] section of the query, you will have to choose another school to discuss. Discuss the school's characteristics that make it a top choice, and then finish by relating these characteristics back to the school where you are interviewing (again, assuming this is the school the interviewer mentioned in the question).

That's it for this straightforward Chapter 21. Brainstorm and practice your school specific questions then get ready to put your salesman hat on for Chapter 22.

Category XVII: Sell Yourself

Selling yourself is what a medical school interview is all about. While most questions allow you to subtly display your positive qualities and experiences, these "sell yourself" question are literally asking you to show off. It's time to be a salesperson.

Q154: *What do you want me to say about you to the admissions board?*

A154: This question offers the perfect opportunity for you to summarize your strengths and the reasons you will make an excellent addition to the medical school class. I like using the rule of three here, as it will help the interviewer remember exactly what to present to the admissions committee. For example,

> "I'd like you to tell the admissions board three main things about me: I have a deep-seated passion for serving others through medicine as proven by my years of community service and clinical experiences in both the US and abroad; I am both a leader and team player, as I demonstrated as captain of the university's swim team; and I will add diversity

to this school through my unique experiences working as a teacher in Asia."

As you see in this example, it is best to provide evidence of everything you say. The skills or qualities you mention should be supported. There are, of course, other ways you can play this question. You may provide a list of your top strengths with evidence or reiterate why you are entering medicine. I've even heard pre-meds make bold statements of response, such as, "I would like you to tell the admissions board that I would attend if accepted" or, "Please tell them I am the best candidate you have ever seen." Said in the right way and to the right interviewer, such candid responses can sometimes go over well. But you have to read the interviewer. I suggest having a formal, more conservative response prepared along with an edgier version to be used in the right setting.

Q155: *Why should we admit you?*
A155: The rule-of-threes answer from Q154 works perfectly here. This query leaves less room for bold answers.

Q156: *What would you like written in your obituary?*
A156: This question is asking you to define a successful life and show the interviewer what you will do with your medical degree. Many pre-meds only discuss how they want to be remembered professionally. While selling the interviewer of your future as a medical professional is important, I believe thinking more broadly about your life provides a better answer. Include what is most important to you in addition to your work, such as family, past-times, travel, *etc.* You may also consider including adjectives (*e.g.,* compassionate, generous, curious, witty) as a way to work in your strengths.

Q157: *How will you change the world?*

A157: I love this question! It's bold and deserves a courageous answer. As no one will check back and see if you changed the world in the exact way suggested, feel free to go for broke. Cure cancer, end malaria, create an affordable medical device that decreases childbirth complications, set up a free clinic in Harlem, devise a policy that leads to true universal care in the US, *etc.* How you choose to change the world tells the interviewer what issues you care about most.

Q158: *Imagine you are on trial and we are the jury. Try to convince us you are compassionate and empathetic.*

A158: Convince through examples. You have already learned to use anecdotes/details/specifics to prove your points. Simply do it again here. You can even lead into your answer with a sentence such as, "Let me provide a few examples to show my compassion and empathy."

We've reached the end of Chapter 22. Instead of plowing ahead after brainstorming and practicing how to sell yourself, take a breather and gear up for a long but fun Chapter 23 that requires thinking outside the box.

Category XVIII: Outside the Box

"Outside the box" questions encompass those queries that seem to come out of left field and are often meant to see how you handle being put on the spot. Though I am a huge proponent of preparation, the best answers to these questions often come from going with your gut and providing the first answer that pops into your head. Honestly, most interviewers will not remember the exact answer to many of these questions. What they really want to see is if you think on your feet or crumble under pressure. When practicing these questions for the first time, don't give yourself time to think. Just answer. I bet you will find that 80% of the time you will have given a strong answer requiring few changes. Of course, if you think your gut response is horrible, come up with something better.

Q159: *If you were a cereal (animal, book, tree, dessert, kitchen utensil, etc.), what kind of cereal would you be and why?*

A159: Many pre-meds answer this by stating their favorite cereal (animal, book, *etc.*), and then struggle with the "why." Your goal is to pick a cereal possessing the characteristics you view as your strengths. I was asked this question and responded, "Wheaties, because it is the breakfast of champions." This was well-received as I was a collegiate athlete. But less punchy answers will do. For example, "If I were a cereal, I'd be Fruit Loops because they are colorful and diverse," or, "I'd be Kashi Lean because it gives people energy and promotes health."

Q160: *What TV character is most like your personality?*

A160: Another question asking you to show your best qualities in a creative way. If one TV character nails who you really are, go with it. But it is ok to choose multiple characters. For example, "I'd say I am a cross between Miranda and Charlotte from the HBO series *Sex in the City* as I am extroverted, career-driven, and not afraid to speak my mind, while also being a good listener and someone people come to for help."

Q161: *If you walked into a room with a block of stone and a chisel and were asked to carve an idea or concept, what would you carve and why?*

A161: Carve anything you'd like. I do suggest, however, that you carve something you know a bit about or want to learn more about, as you will likely be asked follow-up questions.

Q162: *If you were given a million dollars, what would you do with it?*

A162: A million dollars doesn't go as far as it used to, but it certainly would be fun to have it lying around. Here's my answer:

"If I were given a million dollars, I would first have to hand about 50% to the IRS and my state tax authority. Then I'd split $100,000 between my favorite charities, which include Medicine Sans Frontieres to provide healthcare in conflict-ridden areas, a non-profit in Vancouver helping victims of domestic violence gain skills so they can support themselves, and UNHCR to assist refugees. I'd then use the remaining $400,000 to start a business using technology to develop elegant solutions to medical issues in countries where the annual family income is less than $1 a day. And if there was any money left, I'd love to go on a Safari in Botswana."

The exact details of my answer are less important than what they say about me – I understand the realities of tax, support charities that work in austere environments or focus on abuse victims, have a business mind, and love to travel. When crafting your answer, think about what it says about you.

Q163: *If the military draft was reactivated and you were drafted tomorrow into the army, what would you do?*

A163: On the surface, this seems like a simple question. Most pre-meds think you have to say, "Then I'd join the army." But you should go deeper with your response. You do have the right to be a conscientious objector if you are, for example, a Quaker. If this is not your situation and you are not excited about joining the army what else can you say? How about something like,

"Given it is illegal to avoid the draft unless one meets requirements such as conscientious objector status, I would follow the rules and join the army. But as I've never shot a gun and have a hard time with the idea of killing another person, I'd research roles where I could use my leadership and teamwork skills, in addition to my interest in medicine, to help others. For example, I could be a medic or work in health administration or policy."

Notice how I again created a response to highlight my skills? It works every time.

Q164: *What is your favorite book (movie, magazine etc.) and why?*

A164: This should be easy for you. Pick your true favorite (and not what you think the interviewer wants to hear). Don't mention *War and Peace* as your favorite book just to impress if you read it 10 years ago and can't remember many of the details. As with many out-of-the-box questions, the "why" part of the question is the most important.

Q165: *Can you tell me about a book that changed your perspective on life?*

A165: You may use the answer to Q164 if it changed your perspective. If it didn't, then come up with another answer. I'd answer this question with,

> "I just read *The Circle* by Dave Eggers. It is a novel highlighting the pros and cons of companies like Google, Facebook, and Apple and the impact they have on our lives. It made me realize how little privacy we have left these days. While reading the book, I reviewed all of the privacy settings on my Internet and social media services and didn't like what I found. So I made changes to ensure maximum privacy. I now approach all of my online activity with a more critical eye."

Q166: *Who is your idol/inspiration and why?*

A166: I will repeat a theme here: the person you pick is less important than the qualities that he or she possesses. The person may be famous, infamous, a member of your family, or a friend.

Q167: *I work for TIME Magazine and am in charge of selecting the person of the year. Whom would you nominate and why?*

A167: You may be able to use your Q166 response here if the person has done something very special in the current year. If not, think of someone who has. And never forget the "why" part of the answer.

Q168: *If you could have dinner with three people, living or dead, who would they be and why?*

A168: It's amazing how your answer to this question shows what matters most to you. When choosing your three, try and pick people with different strengths and in unique fields; this will highlight your all-around interests. A pre-med who provided my favorite answer to this question took a unique perspective. She focused less on individual strengths and more on how the three people would interact if they all sat down at the table together. Out-of-the-box questions lend themselves well to creative interpretations.

Q169: *Who has been a mentor in your life?*

A169: Webster defines a mentor as "Someone who teaches or gives help and advice to a less experienced and often younger person." Think of someone who is your trusted adviser in any area of life, whether it be professional or personal.

Q170: *Tell me a joke.*

A170: I find this question incredibly difficult as I have a terrible time remembering jokes. If you can believe it, I've answered this question with, "Knock, knock." (Interviewer says, "Who's there?"). "Interrupting cow." (Interviewer asks, "Interrupting cow?"), and I interrupt with a "Mooooooooooo." I know, ridiculous. But it got a laugh and we moved on. Perhaps you'd like to present a joke that is actually funny. Of course, please avoid jokes with lewd or inappropriate themes and absolutely no cursing.

Q171: *Tell me a funny story.*

A171: If you find a joke that is also a funny story, then you have killed two birds with one stone. Otherwise, you need to come up with a funny story. Again, avoid anything that could be taken as offensive.

Q172: *What's the best advice you have ever been given?*

A172: Think of the mentor you discussed in response to Q169. What was the best piece of advice he or she gave you? If that exercise does not lead to a suitable response, turn to your parents and siblings. Did they ever give you great advice? How about a friend? Someone out there has given you guidance you took to heart, and it has changed your life for the better. The best advice I received was, "You can do everything you want in your life, just not all at the same time."

Q173: *What is the most interesting fact you know?*

A173: Here is my answer to this question, "The most interesting fact I know is that kangaroos can put pregnancies 'on hold' until the climate is right for the joey to have the greatest chance of survival." I bet you have a similar random piece of knowledge you'd like to share.

Q174: *Give an example of a time you changed your position on a topic. Why?*

A174: I think the best way to answer this question is to think of a time when learning a new piece of information changed your opinion on a topic. Political and ethical issues work well for this question, but be careful not to offend and always defend your answer.

Q175: *Explain to a six year old how to tie shoes without using hand gestures.*

A175: This is harder to do than you think. Sit on your hands and practice this one. Take into account the concrete thinking of a six year old.

Q176: *Define pain without examples to a six year old.*

A176: Fortunately, you don't need to sit on your hands for this one. But again, you do have to put yourself into the shoes of a child. Use simple, concrete words. For example, "Pain happens when something makes your body go, 'Ouch.'"

Q177: *How would you teach someone who doesn't speak English to use a toothbrush?*

A177: Notice this question doesn't limit your answer to words. So, of course, you have the option of teaching through action.

Q178: *I'm visiting your state/school, and I've never been there before. Where would you take me?*

A178: I'd take the interviewer to my favorite place or my top three locations. As you know by now, explaining why you are taking the interviewer to each location is more important than the actual place.

Q179: *Name five things you can do with a pencil other than use it to write or draw.*

A179: Don't think, just speak. This is the perfect question to answer off the top of your head. Here goes: "Scratch an itch, stake a small plant, play swords, make a fire, use as a hair accessory in a bun."

Q180: *My house is infested with chipmunks. What should I do?*

A180: Interviewers who pose this kind of off-the-wall question want to see how you handle a situation with which you likely have no experience. As with all outside-the-box questions, there is no right answer. The key is to show your thought process out loud. March the interviewer though your proposed solution step by step. I'd probably go deeper than the obvious answer of, "Call an exterminator."

Q181: *Do you ever think about your own mortality?*
A181: Answer "Yes" or "No," and then give a brief explanation for why you do or do not.

Q182: *Do mid-level providers who obtain PhD's have the right to call themselves "Doctor" in a clinical setting?*
A182: Very controversial question. No right answer. Be honest and defend your response.

Q183: *What kind of medical problems will we face on Mars?*
A183: Even if you don't know much about Mars, you can still answer this question. Think about issues that will be faced in an environment very different from our own with respect to climate/distance from sun, access to water, gravity, *etc.*

Whew! We are done with Chapter 23 and Week 4. Once you've finished brainstorming and practicing outside-the-box questions, put the book down and come back tomorrow to review any Week 4 questions that tripped you up. In Week 5, we switch gears and focus an entire week on policy, system, and public health questions.

WEEK 5

We change gears this week to focus on health policy and public health. With the tumultuous passage of the Affordable Care Act (also know as Obamacare or ACA), both the policy and politics of the health system are on the forefront of most doctors' minds. It is a rare medical school interview that doesn't touch on health policy in some form. The topics of public and global health are also fare game in medical school interviews, especially if you expressed an interest in one or both of these fields in your application.

Day 1
Read Chapter 24 (Category XIX: Policy/Health System/Public Health)
Gather resources to increase fund of knowledge

Day 2
Read gathered resources for a minimum of two hours

Day 3
Read additional resources for at least another two hours

Day 4
Brainstorm answers to Chapter 24 questions
Practice answering each question out loud

Day 5

Look up information required to improve your responses and amend as necessary

Day 6

Practice any questions you still find challenging

Day 7

Take the day off

CHAPTER 24

Category XIX: Policy/ Health System/Public Health

Health policy and public health questions make many pre-meds nervous because of the underlying political currents. But though topics such as the Affordable Care Act often create intense feelings in people, you should not shy away from stating your honest opinion. As long as you back up any views with facts and sound reasoning, your interviewer will be impressed even if he or she holds opposite views. Many interviewers will play devil's advocate regardless of their personal opinions to generate an interesting debate during the interview. Sometimes the most divisive issues make for the best interview conversations.

As of this book's writing, the hottest health policy topic is undoubtedly the ACA. You likely have at least a superficial understanding of the ACA from watching or reading the news, but I suggest you do more in-depth research to ensure you can speak in a well-informed manner. You don't need to be a health policy expert, but you should know enough to form an opinion, defend your views with specifics, and give good consideration to the counter perspective(s).

Begin your health policy and public health preparation by organizing resources. Start a paper or virtual file of the articles/videos you find and organize them so you can review them later. Then spend at least two hours reading (and likely more). When something peaks your interest, delve further with more research and reading. I suggest allowing the first three days of this week to reading this chapter, gathering resources, reading articles/watching videos, and performing further research and reading. Here are my suggestions of where to begin learning about the ACA and other health policy/ public health topics:

- For a nice overview of the US healthcare system, read a book like Askin and Moore's *The Health Care Handbook: A Clear Concise Guide to the United States Healthcare System.* As the system is changing before our eyes, be sure to look for the most recent editions of such overview books.

- Head to the Commonwealth Fund website: http://www. commonwealthfund.org/topics/affordable-care-act-reforms. The Commonwealth Fund is a private foundation focused on health policy. It's a great overall health policy resource and dedicates an entire section of its website to the ACA.

- Review newspaper media coverage. Go to your favorite major newspaper (*New York Times, Washington Post, LA Times, Chicago Tribune, Wall Street Journal, USA Today, etc.*) and type "Obamacare," "Affordable Care Act," or another health policy term into the search bar. You will see dozens of relevant articles pop up. Look for summarizing articles explaining the ACA bill in layman's terms and opinion pieces giving one point of view. By reading other people's opinions, you will better be able to form your own.

- Search sources such as *The Economist, The New York Times Magazine,* and *The New Yorker* for longer, often more detailed articles on the Affordable Care Act or other health policy questions. Soak up the details and pay attention to the pro and con arguments given. If you don't wish to pay for these news sources, you can often access them for free at your university or public library.

- From now until the end of interviews, spend thirty minutes a day with your favorite news source, be it network TV news, CNN, *Huffington Post*, or even Twitter. Pay attention to any comments on any health system or public health topic and think about whether or not you agree with the opinions presented. Dedicating 30 minutes a day to current events is a great habit to continue into the future.

- Check out the White House's Affordable Care Act webpage: http://www.whitehouse.gov/healthreform. The site is dedicated to promoting the health reform's successes. Of course it is biased, but it is a useful place to read about the most recent ACA stats. This site will, of course, change with whomever is in power.

After doing your research, form your own opinions. The key to answering most health policy questions is to be knowledgeable, understand multiple sides of the issue, and state your opinion clearly and supported with facts. Of course, the ACA is the current hot topic, but this could change overnight with leadership and legislative changes. Fortunately, the resources listed above will keep you up-to-date on any important health policy topics.

Preparation for public and global health questions is a bit trickier, as the questions tend to be much broader. During your daily, 30-minute news reading, pay attention to public health-related current events, such as natural disasters, refugee crises, and disease outbreaks. You will likely be asked questions about what is in the current or very recent news coverage. For example, if you are interviewing during an Ebola outbreak, be sure you have read widely on the subject.

Q184: *What do you think are the biggest challenges facing the healthcare system today?*

A184: There are so many challenges facing the healthcare system today that you should have many options to choose from. The hardest part will be picking your top three. Here's a list to get your creative juices flowing:

- Creating affordable, high-quality care for all Americans
- Slowing exponential increases in medical costs
- Changing incentives for pharmaceutical companies to decrease drug costs and encourage research and production of drugs to treat a broader range of diseases, especially those affecting impoverished populations
- Training and equitably distributing primary care physicians
- Ensuring medical care is consistently high quality throughout the US
- Facing the challenge of obesity
- Reducing smoking incidence and prevalence
- Treating chronic disease
- Caring for an increasingly elderly population
- Decreasing medical tuition to ensure the most talented Americans have the opportunity to enter the profession regardless of socioeconomic status
- Addressing the medical issues caused by poverty

The rule of threes works perfectly here. I suggest picking your top three challenges and using personal anecdotes to show your understanding of each. Such personal anecdotes may stem from clinical experiences (including when you've been a patient), coursework, travel, research, or even reading on the subject. You can work reading into a response by saying something like, "Last week I read an article by Ezekiel

Emanuel in the *New York Times* that discussed..." Using the author name and source when discussing your reading is more impressive than only mentioning, "I read an article last week..."

Q185: *Where do you see the state of healthcare going over the next 10 years?*

A185: It will be hard to answer this question without mentioning health policy and the ACA. Fortunately, you have already researched the ACA and formed an opinion. Other areas you can discuss are technology, pharmaceutical policy, global health trends, medical education changes, population shifts, etc.

Q186: *How would you fix healthcare?*

A186: There are too many fixes needed to include all of them in one answer. So I suggest picking a few issues you feel strongly about. Do you believe the US should move to a public, universal care system like Australia, England, or the Netherlands? Do you think the key to fixing healthcare is focusing on primary care and preventative medicine? Do you feel reducing the costs of pharmaceutical drugs will make the biggest difference in health care affordability? Are you dismayed by the lack of price transparency in health care? Do you want medicine to be run more like a business? Speak about what you care about most and your answer will come across well, even if the interviewer does not completely agree with you.

Q187: *If you could change one thing about the Affordable Care Act (Obamacare), what would it be?*

A187: Since you have already done your research on the ACA, this will be a simple question for you to answer.

Q188: *Give me three positives and three negatives about the Affordable Care Act.*

A188: You are more likely to be asked, "Give me one positive and one negative about the ACA." But I want you to be prepared for the hardest questions that may come your way. Given you have to provide six responses, initially you don't need to give long explanations for each point. If the interviewer wants more information, he or she will ask for it. For example,

"Three positives are removing pre-existing condition clauses from health insurance, allowing children to stay on their parents' insurance up to age 26, and expanding affordable insurance coverage to over 10 million Americans thus far. Three negatives are insufficient planning that led to difficulties with the roll out, lack of strong focus on cost control, and putting such a large emphasis on expanding Medicaid, a system notorious for very low provider payments and that many doctors won't accept."

Q189: *What do you think the term Obamacare means?*

A189: This seems like a leading question from someone who, perhaps, has a negative view of the ACA. Don't feel you must bash Obamacare if you believe it has positive qualities. I would answer this question by discussing the overall goals of the ACA, and then highlighting some positives and negatives.

Q190: *What do you think about a public option for health insurance?*

A190: A public option for health insurance became a huge topic of conversation during the Affordable Care Act debate. Initially, the democrats wanted a public insurance option to be part of the bill, but it was eventually removed. Basically, a public option for health insurance would involve the government expanding insurance run by the federal government or state, like Medicare or Medicaid, to the general population. Proponents of a public health option often speak of the power of pooling risk, allowing the government to decrease costs through buying power, and creating affordable insurance options. Opponents most often discuss government inefficiency and a slippery slope to a national, government-run healthcare system. Of course, there are many other pros and cons. If you haven't come across this topic in your previous reading, do some more research. An Internet search for Obamacare and public health option will give you plenty of reading material.

Q191: *What do you think about health insurance mandates?*

A191: Health insurance mandates are another popular topic of discussion as a result of the Affordable Care Act. In the ACA, the government made it mandatory for all Americans to obtain health insurance or be subject to a penalty. This issue went all the way to the US Supreme Court, and the mandates were upheld. I suggest answering Q191 by giving both sides first, the pros and the cons, and then stating your opinion.

Q192: *Do you think we should have universal healthcare?*

A192: When answering this question, first define universal healthcare. Some think it implies a government-run health care system, often called a "single payer system." But universal health care could mean everyone having access to a base level of healthcare regardless of payer. Explain what you think the term means, and then give your opinion on whether or not we should have it.

Q193: *If you were president, what would your health reform bill look like?*

A193: Given the ACA has passed and has been implemented, the easiest way to answer this question is to state what about the ACA you would keep or not keep. Your three positives and three negatives about the ACA should help you. If you are well-versed in health policy and have devised the perfect health care system for the US, by all means share it with your interviewer!

Q194: *What do you think accounts for the high cost of healthcare?*

A194: People write their PhD dissertations on such topics, and a 30-minute interview will not be enough time to cover a complete cost analysis of the US health care system. Devise an answer giving three main reasons you think Americans spend the most on healthcare compared with every other country in the world, and yet don't have the health outcomes to show for it. Again, The Commonwealth Fund website (http://www.commonwealthfund.org/) can provide insights here.

Q195: *If the president approached you to help solve a local obesity problem, how would you go about making a difference in the community?*

A195: Begin your answer with what you presume are the main causes of the local obesity problem (such as lack of access to healthy food, education, and exercise options; eating inexpensive "empty" calories; danger of playing outside, *etc.*), and then move to how you would address these causes.

Q196: *How would you recommend alleviating the shortage of primary care doctors in certain areas of the US?*

A196: State the reasons you think we have a shortage in the first place. Then discuss methods to alleviate the problem, such as incentivizing medical students through loan-repayment, increasing Medicare and Medicaid reimbursement schemes to primary care physicians, allowing primary doctors to be paid based on outcomes, guaranteeing jobs to recent residency graduates, promoting primary care in medical schools, allowing foreign-trained physicians to practice in the US without repeating residency, *etc.*

Q197: *What do you think are the three most pressing public health issues facing the US today?*

A197: The hardest part of this question is not coming up with public health issues, as there are plenty, but listing the three you think are most pressing. What issues do you think have the greatest impact on the American population? Examples include: Obesity and its related conditions, rising cost of healthcare despite the ACA, increasing complexity of communicable diseases, poverty, smoking, chronic disease, aging population, gun violence, antibiotic resistance, uneven access to health insurance based on state of residence, expense of healthy food, *etc.*

Q198: *How can we work to reduce the discrepancies in health care delivery in different areas of the city/state/country?*

A198: It is a well-known fact that certain areas of the US have poorer access to healthcare than others. Why do you think this might be? Pick your top three causes, and then discuss how to change/fix/reduce these causes.

Q199: *What are your thoughts on alternative medicine?*

A199: Alternative medicine is now commonly referred to as "complementary medicine" and includes non-traditional medical practices such as acupuncture, herbs, cupping, reike, massage, and hypnosis, just to name a few. Speak about how you see alternative practices and therapies fitting into more mainstream medicine.

Q200: *What technology do you believe will have the biggest impact on healthcare in the next 10 years?*

A200: Many pre-meds answer this question with the latest cool technology but can't explain how it will make a great impact. Sometimes technology that doesn't make headlines has the biggest impact. For example, Plumpy Nut, a food substitute, has dramatically reduced the prevalence of malnourished children in Africa. Conversely, the famous da Vinci surgical robot is flashy but, at the time of this writing, has never been proven to improve outcomes. When answering this question, you may name an already existing technology or one you think will be invented in the near future.

Q201: *What do you think will be the next great global medical breakthrough?*

A201: Notice this question asks you to think globally. A medical breakthrough in the US may not necessarily have a large impact in Latin America or Asia. Answer this question by describing a medical advancement you think will make the greatest impact on the world.

We've reached the end of Chapter 24, which comprises the entirety of Week 5. Once you feel confident about your health policy and public health research, reading, brainstorming, and responses, take a day off, and then move on to Week 6.

WEEK 6

Ethical and behavioral questions have gained popularity in medical school interviews as a means of testing less about your moral code and more about how you think. These types of questions are the mainstay of MMI interviews, but are also increasing in popularity in "traditional" interviews.

Given the number of possible ethical questions is infinite, my goal in Week 6 is to provide you with the resources and framework to answer any ethical question that comes your way. I have found so many pre-meds struggle with answering ethical/behavioral questions that I have dedicated all of Week 6 to research and reading on these topics.

Day 1
Re-read Ethical/Behavioral questions from Chapter 5
Read Chapter 25 (Category XX: Ethical/Behavioral Terms and Strategy)

Days 2-7
Read as much about ethics and behavioral topics as possible

CHAPTER 25

Category XX: Ethical/Behavioral Terms and Strategy

Ethics is a tricky word to define. Inspired by articles from the Markkula Center for Applied Ethics (https://www.scu.edu/ethics/ethics-resources/ethical-decision-making/what-is-ethics/), I think it's easiest to start with what ethics are not. Ethics do not equal religion. Yes, many religions preach the importance of high ethical standards, but ethical behavior is not limited to only religious people. Ethics certainly apply to atheists too. Some ethicists would say that euthanasia, in certain circumstances, is ethical, whereas many religious teachings state euthanasia is immoral. Also, ethics do not equal law. Laws may be based on ethical principles but law and ethics often come into conflict. Slavery and Jim Crow laws highlight this point. Further, ethics do not equal accepted societal behavior. On most issues, it's impossible to determine exactly what is socially acceptable, since views will vary within society. Can you imagine taking an opinion poll on abortion to determine if it is ethical? Nazi Germany is an example of where socially acceptable does not equate to ethical.

So what are ethics and how do ethics relate to morals? Ethics in singular form is a branch of philosophy that studies the standards of right and wrong that dictate what is good and bad behavior. Put another way, ethics tries to answer the question, "What actions are right and wrong in particular circumstances?" In plural form, the word ethics refers to principles that govern a person's behavior. So that's ethics. Now what about ethics vs. morals? I like how the Grammarist makes a distinction between these commonly interchanged words. While ethics are the principles of right conduct, morals are the principles on which an individual's judgment of what is right and wrong are based. Ethics attempt to be objective, shared principles promoting fairness, while morals are more subjective and often filtered through the lens of religion or personal worldview. This is the easiest but likely too simplistic way to thinks of ethics vs. morals: ethics are the science of morals, and morals are the practice of ethics.

When formulating your answers to ethical and behavioral questions, you must consider both the ethics of the situation and how you filter such ethical principles through your own beliefs in religion, law, culture, society, professional standards, *etc.* to create your personal moral beliefs. Given developing a moral code is a highly personal endeavor, medical school admissions committees do not expect a "right" answer to ethical and behavioral questions. They care more about how you come to your answer than the actual answer.

Now that the definition of ethics and the difference between ethics and morals is hopefully clearer, let's move on to defining terms that guide physicians during ethical dilemmas. I have noticed many pre-meds are tripped up when they lack understanding of subtle differences in ethical terminology, such as the difference between euthanasia and physician-assisted suicide/physician aid-in-dying. Thus, I suggest reading up on ethical topics to both ensure you understand the lingo and to help in the formation of your own moral views on medical ethics topics. There are many places you can find information on medical ethics (as a quick Internet search reveals). I find these websites particularly useful:

- University of Washington School of Medicine Ethics in Medicine: http://depts.washington.edu/bioethx/topics/
- Bioethics.net: http://www.bioethics.net/
- NIH Department of Bioethics: http://www.bioethics.nih.gov/
- The Center for Bioethics and Human Dignity: http://cbhd.org/
- PBS Religion & Ethics Newsweekly: http://www.pbs.org/wnet/religionandethics/

Use these resources as the starting point of your ethical/behavioral questions preparation. Focus initially on defining terms, and then move on to reading about how medical ethicists approach individual cases. Take an active approach when reading any piece about ethics. Ask yourself questions such as:

- How did the author define the ethical dilemma?
- What issues does the author site when addressing the ethical dilemma?
- How are principles of ethics filtered through religion, law, culture, *etc.* to create a moral view?
- Are there any issues I think the author has left out?
- Does that author make a persuasive argument? Why or why not?
- How would I address this specific ethical dilemma?

It is often useful to have definitions all in one place, so I have created a glossary of common bioethical and legal terms you may refer to as you practice answering ethical and behavioral questions.

Glossary of Common Bioethical Terms

Advanced directive
Written or oral declaration by an individual capable of making voluntary and informed decisions that indicates preferences for future medical treatments (called instruction directive or living will; *e.g.*, withdrawing life support if in vegetative state) and/or specifies a surrogate decision maker if the individual is unable to make a decision (called a proxy directive or healthcare power of attorney).

Assisted Suicide/Aid in Dying
When a doctor or other individual helps a terminally-ill person kill himself.

Autonomy
An individual's ability to make her own decisions based on her own moral code without coercion or deceit.

Cloning
The act of making an exact copy of a biological entity. Human reproductive cloning aims to create whole individuals. Therapeutic cloning aspires to produce tissues or organs to be used for analysis and/or treatment.

Competence
Used in the setting of an individual being able to make a decision. An individual is deemed competent if he can understand the most important information involved in making the decision, make a judgment about the information, intend and understand an outcome, and communicate wishes.

Emancipated minor

In a medical context, an emancipated minor is free to make her own decisions without consent of a parent or legal guardian. For example, a minor who is pregnant is free to make decisions regarding the unborn child without the consent of a parent or legal guardian.

Embryo

Stage of human development between zygote (first cell formed after sperm fertilizes ovum) and end of eighth week after fertilization.

Euthanasia

Derived from Greek word meaning "good death."

Active euthanasia: Directly causing death (*e.g.*, lethal injection)

Passive euthanasia: Allowing a patient to die by withdrawing or omitting treatment. (*e.g.*, removing from life support)

Voluntary euthanasia: The act of causing death done at patient's request.

Both active and passive euthanasia can be voluntary.

Extraordinary care

Medical treatments that will cause undue physical burden or are unlikely to significantly improve patient's condition and will prolong dying.

Fetus

Stage of human development from eighth week after fertilization to birth.

Hospice

An institution/program dedicated to providing palliative care, specialized medical care for patients with terminal illnesses focusing on quality of life and relief from pain. Hospice services can provide in-patient and home care.

Informed consent
When an individual uses his knowledge and understanding of all relevant information to voluntarily agree to undergo a procedure or participate in research.

Stem cell
A cell that can divide continuously and has the potential to differentiate into various types of cells forming specialized tissue (cardiac, skin, muscle, *etc.*)

Substituted judgment
Legal term referring to making a decision on behalf of someone incompetent to make her own by attempting to determine what that person would have decided were she capable of doing so.

Surrogate decision maker
Individual appointed by the patient (or courts if patient unable) to make medical decisions on behalf of a patient who is incapacitated and/or incompetent.

References:
http://www.bioethicseducation.com/glossary
http://wings.buffalo.edu/bioethics/man-gl-e.html
https://bioethicsarchive.georgetown.edu/pcbe/reports/taking_care/glossary.html

Now that you have a better understanding of ethical terms, it's time to think about how to structure ethical/behavioral question responses. When you are asked an ethical or behavioral question, many thoughts will flood your head. It is challenging to wrangle these ideas into a coherent answer on the spot. So here is an approach that provides your brain with a framework for how to arrange all of your thoughts. I like to call it the "Sandwich Strategy."

Top Layer of Bread

Start by stating the main ethical/behavioral issue(s) posed. In Week 7, I have laid out the questions by ethical category to help you. For example, if you are asked a question about abortion, you may start your answer by saying, "You are asking about my view of maternal vs. fetal rights." By beginning with the overarching theme of the question, you are immediately showing the interviewer your understanding of the main discussion topic. Think of this first sentence as the thesis statement for your answer.

The Meat

Review out loud both or all sides of the debate. You may use the "on the one hand…and on the other hand…" structure or say something like, "There are many sides in this debate I'd want to consider. For example,….," or "Before I speak with the patient, I would first address the following issues…" The key is to think out loud, present your thoughts in logical order, and show the interviewer you see multiple sides of the issue.

The "meat" is usually where you formulate the ethical and moral basis of your answer. When doing so, consider the following documents, organizations, and subjects that guide our moral code:

- The Hippocratic Oath
- The Universal Declaration of Human Rights (1948)
- Religious tenets
- Cultural beliefs
- Societal norms

- Philosophy
- Law
- History
- Academia
- Science

Many interviewers will play devil's advocate and try to pick apart your reasoning. By thinking out loud and reviewing your reasoning in the "meat" of your answer, you will make it much harder for the interviewer to see fault in your argument. Many interviewers believe this part of the answer (*i.e.,* your thought process/reasoning) is the most important.

Bottom Layer of Bread

Directly answer the question. If asked about whether you would provide pills for a patient with terminal cancer to take her own life, be sure to state if you would or would not. Sometimes pre-meds get so wrapped up in stating the ethical dilemma and outlining their thought process that they forget to concretely answer the questions. Directly answering the question often involves stating your own opinion and why you have formed it.

The Sandwich Strategy requires practice because it flips how you answer most questions in a medical school interview. Usually, you'd answer the question in the initial sentence or two, and then provide support in the rest of the answer. But in ethical/behavior questions, I suggest taking a step back and stating the ethical dilemma up front, clearly laying out your thought process, and then directly answering the question.

Before we move on to Week 7, here are a few more tips for use in answering ethical or behavioral questions.

- Interviewers bring their own moral code to medical school interviews. It is not your job to guess their moral beliefs and provide answers to align with their views. Never try to guess what the interviewer wants to hear. Always be true to yourself, defend your views with facts or well-informed opinions, and be ready for interviewers to push you or play devil's advocate. Often times, back-and-forth debate in a medical school interview is a very good sign.

- Put the patient first. In an ethical bind, always remember that Western medical ethics reason it is the patient to whom you have the first responsibility.

- When conflict arises, it is usually best to address, privately and in-person, the individual causing the conflict.

- When stuck on a certain scenario, you can state out loud the need to ask for help from others. Let's say you are unsure of the specific laws in your state regarding the treatment of a child if the parent is refusing treatment. You can tell the interviewer you would overcome this issue by calling the ethics board or risk team at your hospital or the local magistrate to ask for clarification. Similarly, if a patient cannot provide information you require, tell the interviewer you would ask others, such as family, friends, other doctors, *etc.*

- Sometimes assumptions will need to be made to answer the question. It is okay to make assumptions as long as you state them out loud to the interviewer. If you absolutely can't answer a question without knowing a key piece of information, you may ask the interviewer to supply it. Try to avoid this and don't go overboard asking the interviewer multiple questions.

- The "I would" and "If, then" formats often work well in ethical/ behavioral questions. For example, "I would first check to see if the patient had an advanced directive on file. If not, then I would..." You will see how to use these formats in Week 7.

- Feel free to role play. If you are asked to address your patient, Betty, who has come to your office, then you may speak to the interviewer as if she is Betty. Speaking as if you are in the moment can be a very effective technique.

I cannot emphasize enough how important it is to read widely on ethical and behavioral issues. This area of medical school interviews cannot be crammed or memorized. And, more importantly, a healthy understanding of ethical thought will serve you well as a physician, where ethical issues will present themselves regularly. Instead of bemoaning how hard such questions can be, embrace the language and nuance of ethics and the value of developing your own moral compass. Enjoy this week and taking the time to read and think.

WEEK 7

As discussed at the beginning of Week 6, it is impossible to cover every possible ethical or behavioral question you may be asked in a medical school interview. Further, I want you to make an informed decision about your stance on ethics issues and not take the examples in this book as a prescriptive formula for exactly how to answer such questions. Instead, my goal is to inspire you to read more on ethics and guide you on how to ground and structure your answers. Please again note, the example answers are not my suggestions for the "right" way to answer the questions, and they do not represent my own beliefs. The sample answers exist to give you insight into how to approach what can be the most challenging part of a medical school interview.

Day 1
Read Categories A, B, and C
Brainstorm answers
Practice answering each question out loud
Do any research and reading required to better answer questions

Day 2
Read Categories D and E
Brainstorm answers
Practice answering each question out loud
Do any research and reading required to better answer questions

Day 3
Read Categories F, G, and H
Brainstorm answers
Practice answering each question out loud
Do any research and reading required to better answer questions

Day 4
Read Categories I, J, and K
Brainstorm answers
Practice answering each question out loud
Do any research and reading required to better answer questions

Day 5
Read Categories L, M, and N
Brainstorm answers
Practice answering each question out loud
Do any research and reading required to better answer questions

Day 6
Read Categories O, P, and Q
Brainstorm answers
Practice answering each question out loud
Do any research and reading required to better answer questions

Day 7
Practice any questions you found challenging

CHAPTER 26

Category XX: Ethical/Behavioral Questions Practice

In this chapter, I have broken down ethical/behavioral questions into 17 categories (A-Q). As with the previous chapters, you will see significant overlap among questions in each category so that preparing for one question will help prepare for the others. Unlike Weeks 2-5, however, I will not march through the individual strategy or possible answers to each example ethical/behavioral question provided. Instead, I will focus on how to specifically use the Sandwich Strategy introduced in Week 6 to guide your preparation.

Ethical/behavioral questions dig into the core of who we are as humans and deal with intimate, often heart-breaking subjects. The example answers in no way reflect my own opinions and should never be used as a substitute to your own beliefs. As with all medical school interview scenarios, ethical/behavioral questions should be approached with honesty. Your goal is not to get the interviewer to agree with you, but is to be viewed as respectful, compassionate, and well-informed. Please note ethical/behavioral questions responses often require well over the about 60 seconds recommended for most medical school interview questions.

A. Maternal/Fetal Conflict

Maternal/fetal conflict means that what is best for the mother may not be best for the child and vice versa.

Q202: *Would you ever perform an abortion? If so, under what circumstances?*

Q203: *What test(s) would you give to a teenage girl who wants an abortion?*

Q204. *You are caring for a pregnant woman on life support. The child's life is in jeopardy and delivery is urgently needed, but the husband won't agree to the procedure. What do you do?*

Let's start with the Sandwich Strategy. I will abbreviate as follows:

Top Later of Bread (TLB) = main ethical issue
The Meat (M) = issues to consider/thought process/reasoning
Bottom Layer of Bread (BLB) = state your opinion and show how you have formed it. Be sure to answer the question directly.

TLB: The main TLB in Q202-204 is maternal/fetal conflict. Q203 also broaches rights of a pregnant minor, while Q204 brings in the concepts of living wills and power of attorney. Start your answer by stating the overarching ethical dilemmas.

M: The M for Q202-204 may include a discussion of:

- Definition of when life begins
- Rights of mother/father/unborn child
- State/federal laws
- Timing of potential procedures. For example, many states don't allow abortions after a certain week of gestation.
- Person performing the procedure (you vs. colleague)

- Rights of emancipated minor to make medical decisions
- Role/rights of teenage girl's parent(s)/guardian
- Advanced directive/living will
- Power of attorney

BLB: The BLB should include a direct answer of the question supported by ethical concepts.

Let's walk through some example answers to *Q204: You are caring for a pregnant woman on life support. The child's life is in jeopardy and delivery is urgently needed, but the husband won't agree to the procedure. What do you do?* Please note that a very controversial case involving a similar story occurred in Texas to a patient named Marlise Munoz. I suggest doing an Internet search of this case to read about the debate surrounding maternal vs. fetal rights when the mother is on life support.

In the following two example answers, I have put the Sandwich Strategy abbreviations in place to guide you. Of course, you should not include these in your answer.

1. "(TLB) Your question deals with the overarching ethical and legal issues of maternal/fetal conflict, living wills, and power of attorney. More specifically, you are asking me how I would respond to a father who is refusing for his child to be delivered, even though the child's life is in danger, when the mother is on life support and is unable to make decisions. (M) When approaching this situation, I would consider the many ethical and legal intricacies of the case. Given delivery is recommended, I will assume the child is considered viable and is, thus, likely older than 23-24 weeks. Before I met with the husband, I would review if the mother had a living will in place that could guide our care of her and the child. Then, I would determine if she had a

power of attorney designated to make her medical decisions for her if she became incapacitated. This may or may not be the husband. I will assume for the purpose of this scenario that there is no mention of the child in the living will and the husband is the power of attorney. Further, I would research if any federal or state laws exist that could provide insight into the rights of the mother, father, and child in a case such as this. Today, I will assume the local and federal laws do not allow for abortions of a viable fetus but do not speak directly to the issue of a father refusing to have a viable child delivered while the mother is incapacitated. In addition, I would draw on the Hippocratic Oath as it pertains to doing no harm, doctrines of human rights, and my personal belief that the fetus is a life that deserves the care I would provide to any patient. (BLB) Once I had performed these reviews and personal reflection, I would sit down with the father and any family, friends, or religious support he requests to find out why he is refusing the delivery. Once I clarify his reasons and address his specific concerns, he may change his mind and provide permission for me to deliver the child. Should he continue to refuse, I would then contact the hospital's risk department to gain access to the ethics committee and possibly contact the local magistrate to understand my options. These options could include the state taking temporary control of the unborn child or two designated physicians making the decision to deliver the child and override the wishes of the father. After I have done everything in my power to convince the father to give permission to deliver and have confirmed I am allowed to deliver the child by law without his permission, I would deliver the child."

2. (TLB) "You are asking what I would do when the mother of an unborn child is on life support and the father of the child refuses delivery. This scenario involves the legal and ethical issues of maternal/fetal conflict and who has the right to make decisions when the patient is incapacitated, including power of attorney and advanced directives. (M) I will have to make some assumptions to answer this question. First, I assume the father is the legal power of attorney. Second, I assume the mother's advanced directive does not provide guidance for the life of her unborn child. Third, I assume the mother never told her husband or anyone else of her preferred wishes if she was incapacitated and the child's life was in danger, so it could be difficult to follow the principle of substituted judgment. Finally, I will also assume that neither federal nor state laws have exact guidelines for this type of case. (BLB) What I would do in this situation is based mostly on the father's legal power to make decisions for both his wife and unborn child under these circumstances. I would try to determine the basis of his beliefs and ensure he has all of the information required to make a decision. I would also use all hospital resources possible, such as social workers, legal staff, and ethics boards, to review options and ensure the father is well informed. If he still refuses, despite having the facts showing the child will likely die without delivery, I would ultimately feel obligated to respect his wishes, as he is both the legal power of attorney and potential only guardian (if the mother dies) of this child."

B. End-of-Life Care/Physician Aid-in-Dying/Euthanasia

Start to prepare for this topic by reading this excellent description of end-of-life care on University of Washington School of Medicine's Ethics in Medicine website: http://depts.washington.edu/bioethx/topics/pad.html, focusing on the distinctions between physician aid-in-dying (PAD)/physician-assisted suicide, euthanasia, withdrawing life-sustaining treatments, pain medication that may hasten death, and palliative sedation. I also suggest reviewing which states allow for physician aid-in-dying, as this is a hot legislative topic. As of this book's writing, Oregon, Washington, and Vermont have "Death with Dignity" acts legalizing PAD in certain cases.

Q205: *How do you feel about euthanasia?*

Q206: *You are a primary care physician who has cared for Mrs. Mitchell for 30 years. She has been diagnosed with terminal cancer and comes into your office asking for pills she can take when she is ready to die. How do you respond?*

Q207: *Mr. Anderson is dying and in a lot of pain. You want to give him morphine, but the medication will likely lower his blood pressure and hasten his death. You've exhausted all your options. Mr. Anderson is still in pain and wants you to end his life. What do you do?*

Q208: *At what point do you as a physician stop devoting time and resources to a terminally-ill patient?*

TLB: These questions all discuss a different type of end-of-life care issue. While Q205 doesn't need a restatement of the main ethical issue because it is given in the question, you should be able to discern the main ethical issue for Q206 is physician aid-in-dying, for Q207 is euthanasia with the principle of double effect, and for Q208 is end-of-life care taking into account physicians' call to do no harm vs. futility of care vs. sanctity of life in the setting of limited resources. If that last sentence sounded like a foreign language to you, I suggest jumping back to Week 6 and doing more reading on ethical terms.

M: Topics of discussion for Q205-208 may include:

- Patient autonomy
- Patient competence
- Physician call to "do no harm" (professional integrity, Hippocratic Oath)
- Sanctity of life
- Individual liberty vs. state interest
- Compassion
- Potential for abuse
- Passive euthanasia (letting die) vs. active euthanasia (killing)
- Availability of hospice/palliative care
- Quality vs. quantity of life
- Principle of double effect – primary goal of treatment is to relieve suffering but treatment has other effects that hasten death
- Futility of care
- Lack of infinite resources/rationing of healthcare

BLB: Directly answer the question and show how you formed your opinion. For Q205, be sure you have explicitly stated your view of euthanasia and its role in the profession. Should it be legal? Would you ever euthanize a patient? For Q 206, will you give pills to Mrs. Mitchell? For Q207, will you order morphine for Mr. Anderson? For Q208, what criteria would have to be met for you to stop devoting time and resources to a terminal patient?

Here's an example answer using the Sandwich Strategy for *Q206: You are a primary care physician who has cared for Mrs. Mitchell for 30 years. She has been diagnosed with terminal cancer and comes into your office asking for pills she can take when she is ready to die. How do you respond?*

"(TLB) This question is asking how I would respond to a patient who is requesting physician-assisted suicide, also known as physician aid-in-dying. (M) On the one hand, I understand why a patient with terminal illness, who is often losing control of her body, would want to control the circumstances of death. I also appreciate how many ill patients are concerned about pain and suffering and deserve to die with dignity. On the other hand, I believe physicians should do no harm and don't feel comfortable handing out pills with the express purpose of ending life. (BLB) To reconcile these issues, I would begin by telling Mrs. Mitchell how sad I am to hear this news and that she should know I will help her through this challenging time to the best of my ability. I would then try to better understand her motivations and answer any questions that arise. I would then explain that I don't feel comfortable prescribing the pills she has requested as it goes against my physician principles and furthermore is illegal in this state. However, I would make sure she knows of options such as palliative care and hospice that help terminally-ill patients through a focus on quality of life and decreasing pain without overdosing on pills. If she was amenable, I would make a referral to a palliative care specialist and perhaps a psychiatrist who specializes in terminally-ill patients. Most importantly, I would re-emphasize that me not feeling comfortable with physician aid-in-dying does not mean I don't want to be a part of her end-of-life care and that I hope we can walk through this challenging time together."

C. Do Not Resuscitate (DNR) Orders

A DNR order is written by a physician in consultation with a patient/surrogate decision maker and specifies what measures of cardiopulmonary resuscitation (CPR) should be employed in the event of cardiac and/or respiratory arrest. Most DNR orders indicate no CPR should take place. A DNR order is often part of an advanced directive, where an individual states what care she wants or does not want to receive if unable to make decisions.

Q209: *What would you do if you unknowingly resuscitated a DNR patient?*

Q210. *You are an emergency physician caring for a cardiac arrest patient who was brought in by ambulance from a supermarket. As the patient arrives, you receive a call from his daughter stating she has a DNR order and is bringing it in immediately. At the same time, the patient's son arrives in the ED and demands you do everything possible to save his father. What do you do?*

Q211: *A patient who has signed a DNR order has changed her mind and verbally requests you do everything possible to keep her alive. What do you do?*

TLB: No need to get fancy here, as all of these questions bring up aspects of DNR orders. In your intro sentence, define a DNR in your own words.

M: Topics of discussion for Q209-211 may include:

- Patient autonomy
- Advanced directive
- Medical errors/quality assurance
- DNR order theoretically in existence but not physically present

- Identity of medical power of attorney/surrogate decision maker
- Physician's role to primarily respect patient's wishes
- Physician's role to facilitate communication with and between patient's family members
- Patient competence
- Substituted judgment
- Futility of care
- Quality vs. quantity of life

Here's an example answer for Q210. *You are an emergency physician caring for a cardiac arrest patient who was brought in by ambulance from a supermarket. As the patient arrives, you receive a call from his daughter stating she has a DNR order and is bringing it in immediately. At the same time, the patient's son arrives in the ED and demands you do everything possible to save his father. What do you do?*

"(TLB) This question deals with how I would respond to a family disagreement about the end-of-life wishes of a patient who is currently unable to make his own decisions yet reportedly has a DNR order in place that will guide my treatment of the patient in the event of cardiopulmonary arrest. (M) I will assume the patient arrives with CPR being performed by ambulance staff so that my role will be to decide whether or not CPR should be stopped. I will also assume that the daughter told me the specifics of the DNR order, including a request for no CPR or intubation. (BLB) I would begin by ensuring the patient is receiving full care for his cardiac arrest while I sort out the issue. Then, I'd ask the daughter to take a picture of the DNR order and send it to my phone via text/e-mail if she is comfortable doing so. I'd subsequently sit down with the son and ask his reasons for requesting everything be done, when his father reportedly requested no CPR or other heroic measures at the end of his life. During our discussion, I would ask the son to think about what the father would want, and, if I have received a virtual copy of the DNR order on my phone, I would show this to the son and explain that it is a legally binding document. If the son still requests I do everything possible to revive his father, I would bring him into the room where CPR and ACLS were being followed so that he could see first-hand the violence involved and, hopefully, understand why his father did not want such treatment. I would then cease treatment and allow the family time with the patient."

Stop here and brainstorm responses to each question in categories A, B, and C. Then practice answering each question out loud, hopefully recording yourself and reviewing the video. You will likely have to do some research and reading to prepare your best answers.

D. Termination of Life-Sustaining Treatment/Futility

Termination of life-sustaining treatment is often referred to as passive euthanasia. Care is considered "futile" when it has virtually no likelihood of a positive outcome and will only prolong dying.

Q212: *If a patient were brain dead and on life support, how would you make the decision whether or not to discontinue life support?*

Q213: *Would you have "pulled the plug" on Terri Schiavo?*

Q214: *You are caring for a patient you believe has no chance of meaningful survival. The family requests you do everything you can to save her. You have already put the patient on full life support and want to stop with the resuscitation, as you believe the care is futile. What do you do?*

TLB: All of these questions deal with passive euthanasia (withdrawal of life-sustaining treatment) and futility of care.

Some background to get you started with answering Q213. I also suggest you read more on this subject. Terri Schiavo was an American woman who, in 1990, suffered cardiac arrest and consequent severe brain damage. She was deemed to be in a persistent vegetative state, but could breath on her own. After eight years of treatment, her husband petitioned to have the feeding tube providing life-sustaining nutrition removed. Her parents disagreed with the decision. The subsequent case remained in the court system for the next 13 years. Once all appeals of an initial decision to allow the removal of the feeding tube were denied at the federal level, Terri's feeding tube was removed in a hospice center in Florida in 2005. She died 13 days later.

M: Topics of discussion for Q212-214 may include:

- Advanced directive/DNR order
- Medical power of attorney/surrogate decision maker
- Substituted judgment in case of no advanced directive
- Futility of care – concept that doctors have a right not to provide care when deemed futile. Most hospitals require two physicians to make this judgment. Read more about this topic if it is a new concept for you.
- Organ donor status
- Definition of brain death (see American Academy of Neurology definition - http://surgery.med.miami.edu/laora/clinical-operations/brain-death-diagnosis and https://www.aan.com/Guidelines/home/GetGuidelineContent/432)
- Quality vs. quantity of life

- Clear communication with family (it is common to have a family meeting with all physicians and family members present)

Here's an example answer for *Q214: You are caring for a patient you believe has no chance of meaningful survival. The family requests you do everything you can to save her. You have already put the patient on full life support and want to stop with the resuscitation, as you believe the care is futile. What do you do?*

"(TLB) This scenario deals with the issues of passive euthanasia and the futility of care. (M) In this case, I need to consider the specifics of advanced directives, surrogate decision makers, substituted judgment, and my hospital's guidelines for passive euthanasia when care is deemed futile yet the family wants to continue treatment. I will assume the patient is male. (BLB) I would begin by checking with patient's family doctor and family to see if an advanced directive is in place stating his wishes. If in place, I would follow the directive and explain this process to the family. If not, I would see if the patient named a power of attorney or surrogate decision maker. If there is a surrogate decision maker, I would sit down with him and ask what he thinks the patient would have wanted in this situation. If the surrogate decision maker believes the patient would want everything possible done to save him, I would continue with the resuscitation and call in another specialist to the case and obtain a second opinion. If this specialist agrees the care is futile, I would call a family meeting with all physicians, the head nurse, a social worker, and the family to answer all questions and ensure the family understands why we believe the care is futile and not in the best interest of the patient. If the family continues to request full care, I

197

would discuss the case with the hospital's ethics board and risk management team. I would do everything possible to help the family understand my views and feel like they are helping to make the best decision for the patient. It would honestly make me very nervous to withdraw care without some legal backing from the patient or family, though I understand this is sometimes possible with two-doctor authority. Hopefully the hospital's risk department could guide me if it came to this."

E. Spirituality in Medicine/Cross-Cultural Issues

Unlike most interviews where religious and cultural topics are avoided, medical school interviewers often dive into questions of religious and cultural belief and the role they play in medical decision making. If you mentioned a particular religious tradition in your application, the questions are more likely to come up.

While it is easy to enter a debate about religions that are critical of specific medical procedures and practices, I suggest trying to keep your answers positive. You can certainly address the potential areas of conflict, but emphasize the aspects of religion that mesh well with caregiving professions. Further, be careful to not sound like you are "ganging up" on patients who may have religious or cultural traditions that go against your beliefs. Often asking simple questions and ensuring language is not a barrier to communication will lead to common ground in areas of apparent religious and cultural conflict with current Western medical thought.

Q215: *How do you reconcile your religious faith and interest in science?*

Q216: *How do you feel your religious beliefs will influence your patient care?*

Q217: *You are taking care of a child who is seriously injured after a car accident with an actively bleeding spleen requiring a blood transfusion. The parents refuse to consent for the child to receive a blood transfusion given their religious beliefs. What do you do?*

Q218: *A pharmacist refused to give birth control to a patient with a valid prescription citing ethical beliefs. What do you think about this?*

Q219: *If a thoracic surgeon visited his patients prior to surgery and read from his bible to try and "save" them in case any troubles arose, how would you respond?*

Q220: *You walk into the room of a Haitian patient who has had a stroke and is not to eat or drink. The room is filled with his family members who are feeding him and none of them speak English. What do you do?*

TLB: The underlying theme of these questions is a possible conflict of religious or cultural beliefs and current scientific principles.

M: Topics of discussion for Q215-220 may include:

- Your religion's view of accepted scientific principles and theories (there may not be a conflict at all)
- If there is a conflict, how you reconcile it with your own belief system
- Your religion's view of caring for others (many religions hold tenets that say serving others is one of the highest callings)
- Your religion's view of specific controversial medical issues (abortion, birth control, PAD/euthanasia) and your own beliefs in these areas
- Rights of medical power of attorney/parents/guardian
- Rights of minor
- Physician's role to protect the patient while respecting the wishes of power of attorney/parents/guardian
- Physician's role to do no harm when withholding care could have life-threatening consequences
- Patient autonomy

- Rights of medical provider (pharmacists are also providers) to exercise religious or ethical beliefs
- Use of religion as a form of treatment – *i.e.*, a belief in the healing power of prayer in many religions

Instead of providing you with example answers to spirituality in medicine/cross-cultural issues questions, I will provide you with some background to approach Q217 from my own experience. *Q217: You are taking care of a child who is seriously injured after a car accident with an actively bleeding spleen requiring a blood transfusion. The parents refuse to consent for the child to receive a blood transfusion given their religious beliefs. What do you do?* This kind of case occurs more often than you might think, but is usually less dramatic. It is well known that Jehovah's Witnesses believe blood transfusions are taboo, which is why this scenario is common in medical school interview questions. But other, less commonly known religious beliefs can also affect care. For example, Christian Scientists often try to avoid utilizing modern medical care while Scientology teaches its disciples to avoid traditional psychiatric treatments. I often have dealt with such issues in my practice as an emergency physician, and my experience has been that most parents, when they truly understand their child is in significant danger, will agree to a life-saving medical treatment, even if it is technically against their religious beliefs. I think the keys to answering this question are:

1. Letting the parents know you respect their beliefs
2. Clearly explaining all options and what will most likely happen if a blood transfusion is not given
3. Allowing the parents to feel fully supported (as opposed to bullied or ganged up on) with the presence of family and religious leaders.

If, for all of your excellent communication skills, the interviewer states the parents refuse the transfusion and the child will die without it, you do have an option. Every state has a magistrate on call 24 hours a day. If she agrees the parents are not making the best decisions for a minor, she can legally transfer guardianship from the parents to the state. Then, the physicians (often two physician signatures required) can proceed with treatment. This removal of guardianship is usually temporary. Of course, this is a drastic path to follow, but it is sometimes required.

I suggest pausing here to brainstorm answers to each of the questions in categories D and E. Then, of course, practice, practice, and practice.

F. Truth-Telling and Withholding Information

Most pre-meds assume it is never appropriate to lie or withhold information from patients. Medicine, however, is not always that black and white. Use these questions to show you understand the nuances required to be a great physician.

Q221: *Would you ever lie to a patient?*

Q222: *Describe a time when you thought it was better to be dishonest than to tell the truth.*

Q223: *Mrs. Chang is an 80-year-old Asian woman who was hit by a car and is seriously injured. You are the ICU doctor in charge. As you enter Mrs. Chang's room to tell her the diagnosis, her son stops you and requests you do not to tell her the diagnosis as it will be upsetting and prevent her from getting better. He will make all of the medical decisions. What do you do?*

Q224: Is it acceptable for physicians to modify medical information on insurance forms so companies will be more likely to reimburse patients?

TLB: These questions deal with the notion of truth telling in clinical settings as influenced by cultural beliefs and health system challenges.

M: Topics of discussion for Q221-224 may include:

- Concept of paternalism in healthcare
- Patient's right to be told the truth and be the primary decision-maker in care
- Patient's right to request not to be given all information, perhaps for cultural, religious, or mental health reasons
- Patient's capacity to make decisions
- Identification of power of attorney should the patient not have the capacity to make decisions or requests not to know certain information
- Physician's role to do no harm
- Medical fraud
- How best to help patients in a flawed medical system
- Communication with insurance company

I'd like to discuss two of the questions in this category. First, *Q223: Mrs. Chang is an 80-year-old Asian woman who was hit by a car and is seriously injured. You are the ICU doctor in charge. As you enter Mrs. Chang's room to tell her the diagnosis, her son stops you and requests you do not to tell her the diagnosis as it will be upsetting and prevent her from getting better. He will make all of the medical decisions. What do you do?* This is a relatively common scenario in medicine. Most pre-meds immediately jump to an answer detailing patients' rights to know everything about their medical care. But this view of patients' rights tends to be a modern, Western view. Many cultures believe a person who is ill should not be burdened with medical decision making. And, sometimes, patients are too sick to understand. I think the key to this question is to ask the patient. Assess whether Mrs. Chang is well enough to understand the diagnosis and its implications and, if she is, ask her how much she wants to know. If she says she wants to know everything, the son's request will have little weight. If she says, "Tell my son," which is a common response, then go ahead and respect both the patient's and the son's request. Remember, patients have both the right to know and to request not to know. Also, this would be a great question to role play and pretend you are speaking directly with the son.

Second, Q224: *Is it acceptable for physicians to modify medical information on insurance forms so companies will be more likely to reimburse patients?* I want to discus this question because, unlike most ethical/behavioral questions, I think it has a "right" answer in a medical school interview setting. In a world where insurance agencies often deny reasonable claims and prevent doctors from ordering tests they think are best, many physicians face the decision of whether or not to blur the truth to help patients obtain coverage for tests and procedures. It's a bit like Robinhood stealing from the rich to help the poor, with doctors stretching the truth to help patients fight the big bad insurance companies. Unfortunately, such behavior is technically medical fraud, a very serious offense. If you can come up with an instance when modifying medical information to help a patient gain reimbursement from insurance companies is ethical and legal, I'd love to hear it. Because on this question, I don't think there is a strong argument that can be made defending fraud. However, you may consider pointing out that there are times when incorrect codes have been entered accidentally or a correct code has been overlooked and fixing such issues may result in coverage.

G. Professionalism

Professionalism has become a buzzword in medical school admissions. Interviewers want to ensure you will be a student and future physician who will act in a manner suitable for the "noble" profession.

Q225: *How should we deal with "bad" doctors?*

Q226: *If your attending came into work intoxicated but still performed his work well, would you report him?*

Q227: *You are a first year med student. At a party one of your classmates has six beers in one hour and gets really drunk. He behaves similarly at the next party and ends up punching someone. How would you handle the situation?*

Q228: *If your classmate had to miss a class and asked you to sign him in for credit, what would you say to him?*

Q229: *Assume your hospital has regulations about the number of hours you can work per day, and you have already worked the maximum number of hours allowed. What would you do if one of your patients coded at the end of your shift?*

TLB: At the core of each of these questions is the idea of medicine being a profession that requires its members abide by a certain code of conduct.

M: Topics of discussion for Q225-229 may include:

- What is the definition of a bad doctor? Poor outcomes? Not following evidence-based medicine? Negligence? Low patient satisfaction scores? Unusual ordering and treatment patterns?
- Who should police medical personnel? Individual hospitals? State medical boards? Federal government? Specialist boards?

- Punishment vs. rehabilitation
- Do the means justify the ends or do the ends justify the means?
- Physician responsibility to patients, staff, and profession as whole
- Physician as role model
- Do lies have different weights – *e.g.* are there such things as "white" lies or little lies?
- Breaking regulations
- Working while fatigued
- Physician responsibility to do no harm

Let's discuss Q229: *Assume your hospital has regulations about the number of hours you can work per day, and you have already worked the maximum number of hours allowed. What would you do if one of your patients coded at the end of your shift?* Ninety-nine percent of pre-meds answer this question with an emphatic "I'd stay," thinking it is a badge of honor to stay late. If this was the first thought that jumped into your mind when reading the question, take a step back and think about the nuances of the situation. In the following example answer, notice how the Sandwich Strategy is used, but most of the time of spent on the BLB. Don't feel obligated to conform every ethical and behavioral question answer into the Sandwich Strategy approach. As long as you state the main issue (assuming it is not already stated in the question), describe your reasoning, and answer the question, you will likely create a strong answer.

> "(TLB) I understand the point of work regulations. They exist to safeguard patients against errors that can occur when physicians are fatigued and protect residents against potentially unhealthy work situations. (M) But I do think there are situations where it's more important to follow the spirit of the law than the letter. My main goal is to put the

health of the patient first. (BLB) If my patient coded after work hour regulations were exceeded, I would stay, as I assume I have in-depth knowledge of the patient that could be useful. But I would not run the code or perform any procedures, given I am likely quite tired. I would stay and assist by providing the patient's history and medical course when helpful. I would leave as soon as I felt the next team had a solid understanding of the patient's background and could take over care. If the patient passed away, I would ensure the family received support from social work and any appropriate colleagues before leaving."

H. Doctor-Patient Relationship

It's hard to gauge the future bedside manner of a pre-med through an interview. However, certain interview questions try to glean how you will treat patients, especially in difficult situations. The questions below may seem varied, but they all come back to the same question of how a doctor treats patients, particularly in settings of possible conflict.

Q230: *How would you deal with a patient who is non-compliant?*

Q231: *The state where you are practicing passes a law requiring you to ask the citizenship status of all of your patients, and then turn this information into the state at the end of every month. What do you do?*

Q232: *Would you treat an illegal alien?*

Q233: *What do you think about pharmaceutical direct advertising to physicians? To patients? (TV ads, radio ads, mailings, etc.)*

Q234: *A woman with chronic pain and known narcotic addiction presents in your office requesting medications. She refuses to leave until you give her narcotics. What do you do?*

TLB: Each of these questions deals with an aspect of potential conflict in the doctor-patient relationship, such as a patient not following doctor's recommendations, breaches of confidentiality, rights of patients who technically have broken the law, influences of outside industries, and demanding patients.

M: Topics of discussion for Q230-234 may include:

- Potential reasons for patient non-compliance, including:
  Behavioral modification is difficult
  Physician's responsibility to ensure patients understand treatment plans
  Challenge of explaining complex medical issues in terms patients can understand
  Barriers due to language, cultural differences, religious beliefs, *etc.*
  Access/cost issues
  Patient motivation required for most successful medical treatments
- Relevance of citizenship status in patient care
- Does government have the right to know the citizenship status of patients?
- How will citizenship status be obtained (de-identified?) and used?
- Physician's responsibilities to patients/Hippocratic Oath
- Outside influences impact on doctors' prescribing patterns
- Outside influences impact on patients' expectations
- Interesting fact – only the US and New Zealand allow TV pharmaceutical advertising directly to patients and the community
- Who should be responsible for educating patients on most effective drugs and treatments?

- Lack of US national authority to determine which pharmaceuticals are most effective and cost effective (this authority exists in most countries with universal health care systems)
- Physician's responsibility to treat pain yet do no harm
- Epidemic of narcotic addiction in US
- State and federal laws governing prescriptions of narcotics
- Availability of pain specialists
- Availability of non-narcotic pain medications

With the recent public health focus on narcotic abuse and changes to the laws surrounding the prescription of narcotics in the US, I will give an example answer to *Q234: A woman with chronic pain and known narcotic addiction presents in your office requesting medications. She refuses to leave until you give her narcotics. What do you do?* Please note, this query frequently leads to follow-up questions, and the scenario usually ends with the patient becoming belligerent. This is another question where role playing could work well.

> "(TLB) This scenario raises the issue of conflict in the doctor-patient relationship as it relates to the prescription of narcotic pain killers. (M) In dealing with this situation, I'd consider the patient's diagnosis, treatment history including previous narcotic prescriptions, if she has ever seen a pain specialist, the state and national laws governing narcotic prescriptions, and the consequences of giving a prescription of narcotics to a patient I believe is addicted. I will assume she is in chronic pain, has a documented history of narcotic abuse, and has not seen a pain specialist. I will also assume the law supports my right to refuse a patient a narcotic prescription. I've seen similar situations while working as a medical scribe in the emergency department and learned that it is sometimes necessary for medical staff to set clear boundaries with patients, even if

these boundaries create conflict within the doctor-patient relationship. (BLB) After being asked for narcotics, I'd start by reminding the patient that I understand she is in pain, and I want to treat her pain. I'd then explain why I think narcotics are not the best solution for her, especially given we both know she is likely addicted to narcotics, which is a normal physiologic response to using high doses of them. I'd then say that I believe it is unethical for me to provide narcotics to someone addicted to and possibly abusing the drug. I'd finish by reviewing her options, including referral to a pain specialist and non-narcotic pain medication. Ultimately, if the patient refuses to leave or becomes abusive to myself or staff, I'd call security to help with the situation."

Stop here for today and brainstorm your answers to the queries presented in categories F-H, then practice answering each question out loud. Be sure to read up on any topics of which you are unfamiliar.

I. Refusal of Care/Parental Decision Making

Refusal of care/parental decision making questions generally involve patients or parents not following doctors' recommendations. In current Western medical practice, patients have the right to refuse care, as long as they are deemed capable of making decisions. This issue gets more complicated when parents refuse care for their children, as we have seen in the spirituality in medicine/cross-cultural issues category. Remember, you will usually have access to a social worker, government magistrate, and/or ethics board to assist in refusal of care situations.

Q235: *How will you handle a patient refusing treatment you have recommended?*

Q236: *A 13-year-old girl is diagnosed with Hodgkin's. Her parents refuse what you believe is life-saving treatment for her and decide to travel out of the country for alternative, experimental therapies. What do you do?*

Q237: *A seven-year-old boy has presented to your emergency department for the sixth time this month, and you find out his mother has been neglecting to give him his meds. What do you do?*

Q238: *Should it be legal to force someone, who has shown signs of harming himself or herself or someone else, to take medication?*

Q239: *You are seeing a patient with kidney failure who refuses dialysis. He later loses consciousness, and his family requests that you dialyze immediately. What do you say and do?*

TLB: All of these questions revolve around the concept of refusal of care, either by the patient, parent, or power of attorney.

M: Topics of discussion for Q235-239 may include:

- Reasons for refusal or non-compliance
- Patient's decision-making capacity
- Parents'/guardian's/power of attorney's decision-making capacity
- Patient's right to refuse care
- Rights of parents/guardian/power of attorney
- Rights of minor
- Doctor-patient-parent relationship/communication
- Physician's role to protect patient while respecting wishes of parents/guardian/power of attorney
- Suicidal ideation/homicidal ideation thought to be signs of mental illness
- State-based laws allow for the rights of certain mentally-ill patients (one who is a harm to self, harm to others, unable to

care for self/gravely disabled) to be revoked for a temporary period, generally 72 hours, then a legal proceeding is required

- Physician's role to protect patient while doing no harm
- Advanced directive
- Substituted judgment

I'd like to discuss *Q238: Should it be legal to force someone, who has shown signs of harming himself or herself or someone else, to take medication?* because it brings up legal issues you should be aware of and read more about. As stated in the potential topics of discussion for the "meat" of your answer, states have created laws allowing certain medical personnel (generally physicians but sometimes emergency medical system (EMS) personnel as well) to revoke a patient's rights if he is deemed to want to harm himself or others or is thought to be gravely disabled and unable to care for himself. These laws are often referred to "psychiatric holds." This is a big deal. It means certain medical personnel can legally remove rights from a patient for a temporary period of time, usually 72 hours. The patient loses the right to make his own decisions – be it leaving the hospital, taking medications, having visitors, communicating on the phone/ e-mail, *etc*. In most cases, a proceeding must be held by a judge to determine if the hold should be continued or if the patient's rights are re-instated after this 72-hour period. Thus, in a situation where a patient is deemed at a risk of harming himself, it is legal to force him to take medications. Whether or not this is ethical is another story. The question asked about legality, so be sure to give your opinion on whether or not it should be legal. But feel free to take the discussion into the ethical realm. As discussed in Week 6, sometimes legal does not equal ethical.

J. Confidentiality

Patient confidentiality has long been an important part of the doctor-patient relationship. With the passage of the federal Health Insurance Portability and Accountability Act (HIPPA) in 1996, confidentiality of medical records officially became a critical part of patients' rights. In basic terms, a patient has the right to determine who has access to her medical information and medical professionals are expected to protect this right.

As with many ethical issues, patient confidentiality and the related topic of mandatory reporting have a legal footing. As is common in the US, the laws are not consistent in every jurisdiction. For example, certain states have mandatory reporting laws of sexually transmitted or other infectious diseases. Laws also exist allowing for doctor-patient confidentiality to be broken in instances where another person is at risk. There is no need to learn the laws in every state for a medical school interview, but you should understand that the laws vary and bring this up when relevant. The University of Washington Ethics in Medicine website has a great article on the ethical and legal concept of patient confidentiality: https://depts.washington.edu/bioethx/topics/confiden.html.

Q240: *If your sister's boyfriend came to your practice with a STD, what would you do?*

Q241: *The son of a patient is a physician and calls you to discuss his father's case. What do you say?*

Q242: *You are caring for an unconscious patient unable to provide consent regarding release of information to his family. His brother calls you to ask how the patient is doing. What do you say?*

TLB: The key buzzwords for these questions are patient confidentiality.

M: Topics of discussion for Q240-242 may include:

- Patient confidentiality
- Right of patient's partner to know information that could affect her health
- Patient's right to determine who receives information about his health
- Medical power of attorney
- Doctor-patient-family communication

The most attention-grabbing of these questions is *Q240: If your sister's boyfriend came to your practice with a STD, what would you do?*, so let's discuss this one. In this setting, your sister's boyfriend is assumed to be your patient, and thus, has a patient's right to confidentiality. Of course, this doesn't mean you cannot counsel the patient to inform all sexual partners of the STD so they can be tested. In most states, STDs are considered "mandatory reporting," which means you have to tell the state health department of the test results, including the patient's demographic information. Most states have statutes protecting the confidentiality of this information and making it illegal to use the information in court. However, most states also have provisions allowing public health officials to use the information to prevent the spread of infectious disease, such as informing people who have potentially been infected. This is often done without telling the person possibly infected of the source's personal details. Though a state public health officer may have the right to inform someone of her possible exposure to a STD, you as a physician in this scenario likely do not have a legal right in most states to tell your sister. But this doesn't mean you can't be creative, within the law, with trying to find a way for someone to tell her. This scenario highlights the importance of physicians understanding the nuance of laws and possessing strong communication skills.

K. Care of Minors/Emancipated Minors

Care of minors is another legal-heavy topic. Most of the time, the law considers minors unable to make medical decisions on their own. However, there are certain situations where physicians are not legally mandated to obtain parental or guardian consent for medical treatment. These vary by state, but generally include:

Emancipated minor

The definitions of "emancipated minor" are similar in most states. In general, the minor must be 16 years of age, live apart from parents/guardian, and be self-sufficient financially. Some states consider full-time military service and marriage to be adequate grounds for emancipation.

Mature minor

There is no one definition of a mature minor and the decision must be made in family court. A minor may go to court and prove he has the maturity to make independent decisions. If granted, this minor may bypass state laws requiring minors to obtain consent for procedures such as abortion.

Emergency situation

In an emergency situation, physicians have the right to proceed with life-saving treatment without parental/guardian consent (for example, if parents cannot be reached).

Sexual health

Minors have the right to make decisions about their own sexual health, including contraception, testing/treatment for sexually transmitted diseases (STDs) and, in some states, abortion. Further, if a minor has a child, she has the right to make health decisions for herself and the child. But she is not considered emancipated for other types of decisions, such as entering into contracts. Read more about this topic if it is new to you.

Q243: *A 16-year-old female, whom you have known and treated in addition to her family for 10+ years, comes to you asking for a birth control prescription. How do you handle this?*

Q244: *A 13-year-old boy presents with "leaking" from his penis, and you diagnose him with a STD. He begs you not to tell his parents. What do you do beyond prescribing him the correct medication?*

Q245: *A 15-year old girl with a two-year-old child presents with a broken arm and requires surgery. The 15-year-old's guardian is not available to consent for the surgery. What do you do?*

TLB: These questions deal with the concepts of minors' rights to make their own health decisions in certain situations, patient confidentiality, and parental notification.

M: Topics of discussion for Q243-245 may include:

- Rights of minors in certain circumstances to make own health decisions
- Rights of parents/parental notification laws
- Rights of doctors to make decisions for children in emergency situations
- Rights of a minor who has had a child
- Rights of the guardian of a minor who has had a child
- Confidentiality
- Doctor-patient-parent relationship/communication between patient and parents

Here's an example answer for 244. *Q: A 13-year-old boy presents with "leaking" from his penis, and you diagnose him with a STD. He begs you not to tell his parents. What do you do beyond prescribing him the correct medication?*

"(TLB) This scenario involves many ethical and legal concepts including patient confidentiality, the rights of a minor to make decisions about his own sexual health, parental notification, rights of sexual partners to be notified if at risk, and communication within the doctor-patient relationship. (M) I understand there is significant variation in federal and state laws regarding when it is legal or even mandatory to break patient confidentiality. Hopefully, I will already be familiar with the laws in my specific location regarding when it is legal to break patient confidentiality to speak with parents, sexual partners, and the health department regarding a patient. I'd also need to understand the rights of minors regarding their own sexual health. For this case, I will assume a few things. First, that minors have the right to make their own decisions regarding sexual health and that parental notification in these cases is not mandatory. Second, that my state requires mandatory reporting of STDs to the health board, but does not require reporting to sexual partners or parents. (BLB) In this case, I would begin by explaining to my patient that I am not here to judge but to keep him safe. Then I'd discuss the significance of the diagnosis, importance of the treatment, and how to practice safe sex. I'd also want to ensure the sexual act was consensual and he had not been a victim of abuse. Once I am convinced he understands the diagnosis, treatment, and appropriate preventative measures and that he was not abused, I would discuss how I am obligated to report the STD to the health board but not to tell his parents or who he has had sex with. However, I would try to persuade him of the importance of being honest with his sexual partner(s) so they can get tested and treated and of why it's important to be honest with his parents. I would also offer to be present when he notifies his sexual partner(s) and/or tells his parents. In the end, I would emphasize that he can speak to me about any issue he has and educate him about patient confidentiality as it pertains to certain issues. I think it's very important he feel comfortable seeking treatment from me in the future."

Take the remainder of your interview practice time today to research the topics discussed in categories I, J, and K and then do your usual brainstorm and practice sessions.

L. Informed Consent

Let's remember our definition of informed consent: It occurs when an individual uses her knowledge and understanding of all relevant information to voluntarily agree to undergo a procedure or participate in research. These questions tend to blend into other ethical categories, such as care of minors.

Q246: *A three-year-old female arrives in your emergency department unresponsive and with unstable vital signs. There is no adult available to consent for life-saving treatment. What do you do?*

Q247: *As a medical student, you are asked to consent an elderly woman for a hernia repair. She can barely hear and you are fairly confident she didn't understand the consent. When you tell the senior resident of your issue, she says, "Just get it done." What do you do?*

Q248: *Your patient requires gallbladder surgery and speaks only Thai. You do not speak Thai, and there are no interpreters available in the hospital. What do you do?*

TLB: Barriers to informed consent lie at the core of all of these questions. Q246 also involves treatment of a minor in an emergency situation when parental consent cannot be obtained.

M: Topics of discussion for Q246-248 may include:

- Definition and importance of informed consent
- Treatment of minors in emergency situations
- Doctor-patient-parent relationship
- Communication issues (hearing, language barrier, cultural differences)
- Availability of medical power of attorney
- Use of technology to help with communication challenges

A common scenario is presented in Q247: *As a medical student, you are asked to consent an elderly woman for a hernia repair. She can barely hear and you are fairly confident she didn't understand the consent. When you tell the senior resident of your issue, she says, "Just get it done." What do you do?* Medical providers are frequently in a rush and want things to get done quickly. But, of course, they need to get them done right. Notice in this example answer how the M and BLB have been merged and the effective use of the "if, then" approach.

> "(TLB) This questions brings up the issue of informed consent when a communication barrier is present. (M and BLB) I'd start by visiting the patient's nurse to see if the patient wears a hearing aid and ensure it is functioning. If that doesn't fix the problem, I'd try a trick I've seen before – putting my stethoscope ears into the patient's ears and talking into the bell. If I can find no way of making her hear better or if I believe when she does hear properly that she does not have the capacity to make medical decisions, I would investigate

her medical power of attorney/next of kin. If she does have a medical power of attorney, I would obtain informed consent from him. If none of these strategies work, I would return to my senior resident, report my actions, and discuss the possibility of other available options. As I understand both the legal and ethical importance of properly obtaining informed consent, I would not force the patient to sign the document if I didn't think she understood. I know my senior resident may have a negative reaction if I don't get the job done, but I wouldn't feel comfortable compromising the ethical and legal concept of informed consent just to please a superior."

M. Medical Errors

The 2000 *To Err is Human* report by the Institute of Medicine made error reduction by medical providers a top priority. Though a few of these questions don't fit the typical ethical/behavioral format, you can still use the Sandwich Strategy we have discussed. The keys are to clearly describe your reasoning and directly answer the question.

Q249: *How do you think we can decrease medical errors?*

Q250: *Do you think the US should have a national medical errors database? Why or why not?*

Q251: *Medical mistakes are common but not always important. Significant errors leading to morbidity, such as leaving a sponge in the abdomen after surgery, must be disclosed to patients. Should physicians also disclose less important mistakes, such a single inconsequential medication error?*

Q252: *What do you think about the current state of malpractice in the US?*

TLB: The main issues in these questions are self-evident, so no need to repeat them in your answer.

M: Topics of discussion for Q249-252 may include:

- Mandatory, anonymous reporting systems
- Checklists
- Continuing medical education (CME)
- Formal quality assurance programs
- Whose job it is to police "bad" doctors?
- Anonymity of medical error database
- Administrative burden of medical error database
- Access/privacy rules of medical error database
- Mandatory vs. voluntary entry into medical error database
- Use of medical error database information
- Honesty in medicine
- Patient safety
- Malpractice as deterrent to negligent care
- Patient's right to be remunerated for negligent care
- Malpractice as cause of over-testing, which may lead to harm
- Malpractice as cost to physicians and hospitals
- Other malpractice models

Let's discuss *Q252: What do you think about the current state of malpractice in the US?* because it gives us an opportunity to learn more about malpractice system options. Most pre-meds will indicate they are not thrilled with the current state of malpractice in the US, but the key to impressing an interviewer is showing you actually understand the system and its alternatives through your answer. There are many other options for dealing with malpractice issues, including government-funded, no fault insurance; caps on remuneration; and binding arbitration. If you'd like to do some research on a government-funded, no-fault system, check out this Commonwealth Fund article on New Zealand's Accident Compensation Corporation: http://www.commonwealthfund.org/publications/in-the-literature/2006/

feb/no-fault-compensation-in-new-zealand--harmonizing-injury-compensation--provider-accountability--and. Here' an example answer:

> "(No need for TLB) (M) When I hear physicians discuss the current malpractice system, it is often in a negative light. But I think it's important to step back and consider why such a system is in place. I believe the ideal malpractice system would compensate those injured by medical errors and work to prevent such mistakes. While another role could be to deter negligent care, I am uncertain if any malpractice system has ever been proven to do so. I have a hard time believing a doctor who is intentionally negligent will be more so if malpractice didn't exist. (BLB) I think our current malpractice system does aim to compensate those who are injured and this is a positive. But the legal process is an expensive and inefficient one, where lawyers often benefit more than patients. Also, I don't believe it acts as an effective deterrent to negligence and often does the opposite by incentivizing over-treatment because doctors fear being sued. Further, the US malpractice system has no formalized mechanism for preventing errors. It is punitive and not corrective. I think the best model is that practiced in New Zealand, which has no-fault malpractice and focuses on making doctors better as opposed to punishing them. I also like the Kaiser model of binding arbitration, where fellow physicians judge their colleagues work with the goals of improving care and providing fair compensation."

N. Research Ethics

As the Tuskegee syphilis experiment reminds us, research often leads to ethical quandaries. This is why institutional review boards (IRBs) exist to regulate research on humans and ensure ethical and legal standards are met.

Q253: *You are a fourth-year resident performing research and preparing to present your data at an upcoming global conference. Just before you leave, you discover your principal investigator (PI) is falsifying data. What do you do?*

Q254: *Many IRBs stipulate that researchers in developing countries provide the same standard of care for patients as they do in the US. What do you think about this stipulation?*

Q255: *If you could go back in time and ask Henrietta Lacks for permission to use her cells, would you?*

TLB: These questions deal with various aspects of research ethics, including honesty, standards of care in different research settings, and consent to use human cells/tissues for research.

If you don't know who Henrietta Lacks is, then I suggest reading the book, *The Immortal Life of Henrietta Lacks* (http://rebeccaskloot.com/the-immortal-life/). In short, Henrietta was a socioeconomically-disadvantaged African-American woman who suffered from cancer and was treated at Johns Hopkins in the 1950s. Her cells were taken without her knowledge and became known as HeLa, one of the most important tools in the history of medical research. These cells helped develop the polio vaccine, *in vitro* fertilization, and cloning, to name just a few, and they have made many individuals and companies very wealthy. Unfortunately, Henrietta's family never received any compensation for these cells, and they still suffer the effects of significant poverty. Her case raises the issues of informed consent in research and use of human cells/tissues for the good of society and to make a profit.

M: Topics of discussion for Q253-255 may include:

- How to confirm data is being falsified
- How to address those higher up in the medical hierarchy
- Where to seek help (ombudsperson, Institutional Review Board (IRB), medical school dean, *etc.*)
- What standard of care do all people deserve?
- Who is responsible for setting this standard of care?
- Should research be limited if a US standard of care cannot be maintained in a certain setting?
- Is it better to receive substandard care or none at all?
- Should consent be required to use human cells/tissues once they are removed from a body?
- Ownership of human cells/tissues once they are removed from a body
- If money is made from research using human cells/tissues, should the owner be compensated?
- Rights of individual versus benefit to many

Here's an example answer for Q253: *You are a fourth-year resident performing research and preparing to present your data at an upcoming global conference. Just before you leave, you discover your principal investigator (PI) is falsifying data. What do you do?*:

"(TLB) This question deals with research ethics and scientists' responsibility to the medical community, patients, funders, and society to do their best to create truthful findings. (M) When thinking about how I'd handle this situation, I would consider how to prove the data is true or false, how to address the issue with the PI, and whom I could turn to should there be conflict between the PI and myself. (BLB) I'd start by ensuring the data is falsified, whether it be by reviewing the data again or running through it with another member of the research team. If I was sure my PI was falsifying data, I would set up an in-person meeting to discuss my concerns. Instead of accusing my PI, I would state that I had some concerns about the data that didn't seem to make sense and see how he responded. If this in-person meeting did not lead the PI to address the problem by either proving he did not falsify data or admitting to doing so, I'd consider my other options to obtain assistance, such as consulting the university ombudsperson or IRB. With regards to the conference, I would try to ascertain if the entire project had been jeopardized by false data or only certain parts. If I could salvage parts of the project, I would present those. If the entire project was not longer valid, I would respectfully pull myself from the conference agenda."

Stop here to brainstorm and practice the questions in categories L-N.

O. Resource Allocation

Resource allocation is a hot topic of debate in health policy circles. No matter the health care system, there are a finite number of resources that must be allocated. Many health economists therefore claim their discipline is an arm of ethics, as they are interested in how scarce resources can be shared efficiently and equitably such that waste and opportunity costs are minimized and health gain is maximized. But this is where political spinsters have entered the debate and associated certain terms (*e.g.*, "rationing") with "death panels" and supposedly evil, government-run healthcare review boards. These are not trifle matters and often doctors can feel squeezed between generously apportioning resources to an individual patient, knowing that this might mean another patient within the system (perhaps even that doctor's next patient) will receive less. While politicians and policymakers often present as an easy target for criticism in this regard, it is important to acknowledge that they too face the doctor's dilemma, albeit on a larger, more anonymous scale. Because of the politicized nature of resource allocation, be sure to define your terms when discussing the topic.

Q256: *Do you think healthcare should be rationed?*

Q257: *What if while you are spending more time with a terminally-ill elderly patient, you spend less time with a sick child, miss a diagnosis, and the child dies?*

Q258: *If you had $100,000 that could support one cancer patient or 100 healthy patients, how would you allocate the funds?*

Q259: *Of a seven-year-old girl with Down Syndrome, a 35-year-old single man with a former drug addiction, and a 51-year-old man with a wife and two children, to whom would you give a heart if you only had one?*

Q260: *I am the governor, and my wife wants to spend millions on an anti-meth campaign. What do you think about this use of funds?*

TLB: These questions all involve how to allocate finite resources fairly.

M: Topics of discussion for Q256-260 may include:

- Resources are not limitless, including a doctor's time
- Who is or ought to be responsible for resource allocation?
- What constitutes "fair" resource allocation?
- Do certain patients deserve preferential treatment?
- Do the rights of many outweigh the rights of few?
- Do the rights of the sick outweigh the rights of the healthy?

- Role of certain characteristics when determining resource allocations, such as age, co-morbidities, use of illicit substances, *etc.*

Here's an example answer for Q258: *If you had $100,000 that could support one cancer patient or 100 healthy patients, how would you allocate the funds?*:

> "(TLB) You are asking my opinion of how to allocate a finite resource in the setting of 1 cancer patient versus 100 healthy patients. (M) I believe fair resource allocation depends on the specifics of the situation. As such, my answer depends on further information, such as the prognosis, age, and co-morbidities of the cancer patient. I'd argue spending $100,000 to support a 34-year old with intermediate stage colon cancer and no co-morbidities is a good use of funds, while spending this money to support a 90-year old with metastatic liver cancer, diabetes, coronary artery disease, and renal failure is not. (BLB) In certain clinical situations, I do not believe the rights of many outweigh the rights of few and would use the money to treat the cancer patient. But as I said before, my answer would change depending on the specific factors of the cancer patient."

P. Scientific Advancements

Science and technology are progressing so fast these days, it is challenging for regulatory agencies to keep up. This has created an intense debate around the ethics of certain scientific advancements.

Q261: *What do you think about genetic testing for [insert disease name]? (assume non-curable, life-threatening disease)?*
Q262: *How do you feel about stem cell research?*

226

Q263: *How do you feel advancements in gene therapy will affect the future of medicine?*

Q264: *What do you think about cloning?*

TLB: These questions state the ethical dilemma up front and won't require at TLB in the response.

M: Topics of discussion for Q261-264 may include:

- Rights of individual to know genetic makeup
- Psychological ramifications of genetic testing
- Availability of treatment for specific genetic diseases
- Potential use of genetic material/test results in discriminatory manner
- Genetics and heredity of disease (dominant, recessive, *etc.*)/ reproductive rights
- Affect of genetic test results on patient's family
- Source of stem cells (bone marrow, blood stream, umbilical cord blood)
- Potential use of stem cells
- Cost of stem cell research
- Personalized medicine
- Safety and cost-effectiveness of gene therapy
- Medical uses of cloning
- Cloning of humans versus other forms of life
- Cloning of tissues versus entire humans
- Who regulates cloning?

Let's discuss two of these questions. *First, Q261: What do you think about genetic testing for [insert disease name]? (assume non-curable, life-threatening disease)?* Huntington's disease is an example of a condition that could be used to answer this question. It is currently a non-curable, neurodegenerative disease whose symptoms emerge when affected individuals are in their 30s or 40s (often after having children), worsen for 10-25 years, and eventually lead to death. It is inherited in an autosomal dominant fashion. In simplistic terms, this means a child would have a 50% chance of inheriting a disease assuming the other parent is not a carrier. Whether or not to test for such a disease has psychological and reproductive ramifications. Imagine you are currently a healthy 22-year-old applying to medical school (maybe not so hard to imagine). Would you want to know if you are at risk for such a disease, even if you currently don't have symptoms? Why and why not? Discuss these reasons (pro and con) with the interviewer and finish with your final opinion regarding whether or not you think genetic testing for the disease is a good idea.

Second, *Q264: What do you think about cloning?* In this kind of open-ended question, you can provide your answer with structure by discussing the pros and cons of different types of cloning. For example:

> "(No need for TLB) (M) My opinion of cloning depends on what is being cloned. (BLB) The idea of cloning entire humans makes me very nervous, given how easy it could be to use this technology for nefarious purposes, such as making armies. Cloning of human tissues, however, could have a positive impact on health if it is used for such things as creating new organs for transplant. As with many other advances in health-related technology, I think international regulatory boards should be created to closely monitor and police cloning research and implementation and ensure the benefits outweigh the risks."

Q. HIV and AIDS

The history of HIV/AIDS over the last nearly 40 years can be used as a case study of the medical community's response to communicable disease. The virus has been an ethically-, politically-, and racially-charged subject given its means of spread and populations affected. The questions on this subject often speak not just to HIV/AIDS, but also to any disease that is initially untreatable and affects minority and often disenfranchised populations.

Q265: *Would you operate on a HIV+ patient who requires a minor knee operation?*

Q266: *Should we mandate HIV testing?*

Q267: *Do you think money is better spent researching HIV/AIDS treatment or cancer treatment?*

TLB: Though these questions all mention HIV/AIDS, the TLBs vary. Q265 involves a decision to perform a procedure that puts the operator at risk, Q266 brings up the idea of governments demanding citizens be tested for illnesses with public health implications, and Q267 deals with the allocation of limited research funding and the ethics surrounding funding research on preventable diseases.

M: Topics of discussion for Q265-267 may include:

- Rights of patients with non-curable infectious diseases
- Rights of doctors to refuse to provide care that puts them at personal risk
- Likelihood of disease transmission
- Availability of protective clothing to prevent communicable disease transmission
- Rights of an individual to not be tested for a certain disease
- Benefit of population vs. benefit of an individual
- Disease is treatable but incurable
- Availability of affordable treatment and counseling
- Cost-effectiveness and logistics of mandatory testing program

- Allocation of medical research funding, a finite resource
- Should behaviors leading to disease transmission be taken into account for research funding? (*i.e.,* HIV through sex, intravenous drug use (IVDU), and, rarely, blood transfusions; cancer as a result of various factors, including genetics, behavior, and environment)
- Defunding research on diseases contracted through "poor" behavior

Instead of providing an example answer, I will discuss the nuance of each of the questions to help guide your answer. *Q265: Would you operate on a HIV+ patient who requires a minor knee operation?* held more weight when HIV/AIDs was a death sentence and considerably more stigma surrounded the disease. When the HIV virus epidemic started in the US in the 1980s, many physicians refused to treat patients because they did not understand how the disease was transmitted and feared contracting it. This question really comes down to the issue of whether or not you think doctors have the right to refuse to treat patients with non-curable infectious diseases in non-emergent or emergent situations. An interviewer could easily substitute Ebola for HIV. Would you be willing to operate on an Ebola patient?

Regarding *Q266: Should we mandate HIV testing?*, many local and state governments have considered mandating HIV testing in an effort to curb the epidemic given approximately 30% of all infected individuals do not know they are infected and may be putting others at risk. Of course, mandating any medical test will create a debate around individual vs. population rights, availability of treatment and affordable patient counseling, cost-effectiveness, and logistics of instituting and moderating such a program. In your answer, you may weigh the pros and cons of mandating testing (this is a great place to use "on the one hand...but on the other hand), and then state your opinion.

Q267: *Do you think money is better spent researching HIV/AIDS treatment or cancer treatment?* has an underlying message. There have been many objectors to pouring significant amounts of money into finding treatments for HIV because of how the disease in contracted. In a modern addendum, new prophylactic HIV prevention pharmaceuticals are facing opposition for funding with a view they might encourage unsafe behavior. In such arguments, there is often an implication that because the disease is preventable and most often contracted after unprotected sex or IVDU, that research money would be better spent on other diseases contracted by people through no fault of their own. Others argue funding for HIV research should be primarily focused on prevention and not treatment. Still others believe cancer treatment should receive more funding as it is the number one cause of death in the US. But, of course, there is also an argument that cancer often comes about because an individual smokes or does not exercise or eats unhealthy foods. Where do you stand? In the end, I think this question has two important parts:

1. How do we best allocate limited research funds for HIV/ AIDS and cancer?
2. Should the behaviors leading to a disease have any weight in the debate?

This is a very interesting question and worth a good think.

Phew. We have now reached the end of the ethical and behavioral questions section. Brainstorm and practice the questions in categories O, P, and Q. Then spend your last day this week reviewing any questions in Chapter 26 you found challenging.

Though it may be exhausting, preparing for ethical/behavioral questions will make you a better medical student and physician because you will be ready for the ethical situations that inevitably arise. So you aren't just getting ready for medical school interviews here, you are preparing for your medical career.

WEEK 8

Congratulations! You've made it to the final week. Given I am sure you are fatigued from all of the ethical and behavioral questions, we will lighten the mood in Week 8 starting with a focus on unusual interview scenarios, such as group and essay questions, and then moving on to questions to ask interviewers, what to wear, final prep, and post-interview strategy.

Day 1
Read Chapter 27 (Category XXI: Group)
Practice answering questions with others

Day 2
Read Chapter 28 (Essay)
Practice writing an answer to three questions in this book, each in 15 minutes. I suggest choosing one challenge, one characteristics, and one ethical/behavioral question.

Day 3
Read Chapter 29 (Questions to Ask Interviewer)
Prepare three questions to ask potential interviewers for each school where you have received an interview

Day 4
Read Chapter 30 (Style Prep)
Plan your wardrobe for interview day

Day 5

Read Chapter 31 (Final Preparation)
Research your travel plan for each interview
Gather all required documents
Pack your portfolio

Day 6

Read Chapter 32 (Post-Interview Strategy)
Brainstorm whom you would ask for verbal and written recommendations

Day 7

Read any appendices that pertain to you

CHAPTER 27

Category XXI: Group

Group interviews are rare on the medical school interview trail, but it's important to understand the basics of how to succeed in group interviews should one come your way. Begin by reviewing the strategy for group questions discussed in Chapter 3. Then review the following question list.

GROUP QUESTION EXAMPLES

268. You three have just moved into a one-bedroom apartment together. Take 10 minutes to plan out how you are going to live with each other.

269. If you were crashed on a desert island with a group of natives who worship wooden idols, and the pilot has a broken leg that is bleeding, what five items that are common to luggage would you want to have and why?

270. Create a reality show where the winner gets a full ride to medical school.

271. If you were the head of so and so company and we gave you 100 billion dollars, how would you allocate the money?

272. You are on the organ transplant committee and have to chose between two individuals with liver damage who will die if

they don't receive a new liver a) A 35-year-old mother with three children all below the age of six and a history of drug abuse b) A 50-year-old man with 20-year-old twins and a history of alcohol abuse. This person's family has given large donations to the school.

273.   A fourth-year medical student close to graduation messes up (ethically). What would you do to discipline him?

274.   A small town has a sudden surge in DUI and alcohol-related arrests. How would you go about researching the root of the problem?

Yes, many of these questions seem unusual. But they all have the same goal – to see how you work in a group to solve an uncommon problem. Though there does need to be a leader in every group who organizes the brainstorm and presents the group's final answer, that leader does not have to be you. If you are a natural leader and feel it is the best way to showcase your skills, feel free to speak up. But do not step on others toes or, gasp, argue with a member of your group about who will take the reigns. Group interview performance more often sinks interviewees' chances of admission than cinches them. Here are some tips to help you survive the group interview:

- Don't interrupt.
- If you disagree with a point, keep the discussion cordial. A nice tactic is to praise part of the group member's idea before disagreeing with another part of it.
- Say something. If you are introverted and struggle in group situations, you don't need to be the loudest person in the room, but you do need to add to the group discussion in some way.
- Don't repeat another group member's idea as if it is your own.
- Don't hog the floor.
- Encourage others who haven't had a chance to speak to do so.

- If a time limit is given, be sure the group's time is being managed appropriately.
- Ignore the interviewer(s). Focus on the group until presenting the final answer.

The best way to prepare for group interviews is, of course, to practice answering questions together with others. Spend the rest of today trying to wrangle together practice buddies. While fellow pre-meds would work well, your practice mates can really be anyone, from parents to siblings to friends to co-workers. If you can't find anyone with which to practice group questions today, then make it your goal to schedule a practice session.

Have fun with the group questions. How often will you get to work with other smart, interesting people to decide what five items you want to have in your luggage when you land on a desert island?

CHAPTER 28

Essay

Some medical schools include a 10-20 minute (usually 15 minute) essay as part of the interview process. Often, the school will ask you to answer one of three questions. Characteristic, challenge, and ethics questions are quite common. Fortunately, the hundreds of questions you have just read and practiced will prepare you to answer the essay query. However, a verbal answer is often quite different from a written one, so let's review how to tackle the medical school essay question.

Remember the five paragraph essay from high school?:

1. Introduction/Thesis
2. Supporting Paragraph 1
3. Supporting Paragraph 2
4. Supporting Paragraph 3
5. Conclusion

You may use this basic format to answer any medical school essay question. The point of the essay is to see how clearly you state your thoughts in written form, not to determine whether or not you are a great creative writer. Keep the writing simple, tell the reader exactly where you are going, and use specific examples to prove your points.

After you read the question(s), take a few minutes to gather your thoughts and even make a quick outline before putting pen to paper (or words to computer screen). Then begin with a strong thesis statement. Let's say you are asked to write about your three most impressive characteristics. You want to hit the reader over the head with the direction this essay will take with the thesis: "My three strongest characteristics are leadership, perseverance, and passion for making the world a fairer place." Now move onto the supporting paragraphs. The first paragraph will give an example(s) of your leadership, the second of your perseverance, and the third of your passion for making the world a fairer place. End the essay with a conclusion that reiterates the thesis, but vary the words or sentence structure. I know this seems boring and cookie-cutter. But, again, the admissions committees are not looking for a novel. They want to see your thought process. Keep it simple.

Further, the essay doesn't have to be boring. Use examples and details to keep the reader engaged. This is called "showing" as opposed to "telling." Your aim is to use evidence from your own personal experience to prove your point (showing) as opposed to simply stating the point (telling). Which of the two following sentences do you think does the better job of showing as opposed to telling?

1. "Moving up from secretary to vice president to president of Camp Kesem at my university over the last three years has taught me skills including patience, humility, and the ability to make hard decisions even when they are not popular, all skills required to lead my colleagues."

2. "Leaders require patience, humility, and the ability to make hard decisions even when they are not popular."

Obviously, the first sentence does a better job of showing and, thus, makes a more interesting point.

Now let's say you are asked your opinion on an ethical topic: "What do you think about abortion." You can use the five-paragraph essay structure here as well. Notice how I suggest stating your opinions up front in response to an ethical/behavioral essay question, as opposed to using the Sandwich Strategy recommended for verbal responses to ethical/behavioral queries.

Introduction/Thesis
State exactly what you think about abortion and give three reasons for your beliefs. Do not leave your opinion until the conclusion.

Supporting Paragraph 1
Supporting reason 1

Supporting Paragraph 2
Supporting reason 2

Supporting Paragraph 3
Supporting reason 3

Conclusion
Reiterate your thesis

If you'd like, you can also take the "on the one hand, on the other hand" approach to ethics questions:

Introduction/Thesis
State views/opinions/beliefs

On the one hand
What people say who hold views opposed to yours

On the other hand
What people say who hold views similar to yours

Conclusion
Reiterate your views, but vary the words or sentence structure from the thesis statement.

I cannot state strongly enough the importance of using basic essay-writing techniques to approach the medical school interview essay. Keep it simple and answer the questions clearly and succinctly. You will likely only have 15 minutes or less!

I suggest you now choose three questions from this book to practice answering in essay form. Essay queries often come from challenge, characteristics, and ethical/behavioral categories, so I think choosing one question from each of these categories would work best. Set a timer to 15 minutes to recreate the time pressure you will feel on interview day.

CHAPTER 29

Questions to Ask Interviewer

Ninety-nine percent of medical school interviews will end with the query, "Do you have any questions for me?" Many pre-med Internet forums say you have to ask three questions to show your interest in the school. Medical school admissions committee members are busy people. Do you really think they want you to drag the interview on to show interest? The key here is to read the interviewer. If questions flow naturally out of the conversation, go for it and ask away. But if it seems like the interviewer is just being polite, then only ask one question. Ideally, you want to ask a question about something that came up in the interview. If nothing from the interview jumps to your mind when asked if you have any questions, then you may ask questions such as:

- Why do you love it here?
- Would you mind telling me what you like most about this medical school and what you like least?
- Is there anything else you think I should know about [name of medical school where you are interviewing]?
- Do you have any tips for me as I move through my medical education?

- How have you balanced clinical work and research?
- How have you found the new curriculum?
- How did you choose your specialty?

These questions allow the interviewer to speak about their personal experiences and/or impart knowledge. Most interviewers will enjoy the chance to show off their school or play a small mentorship role. Try not to ask esoteric questions the interviewer is not likely to know how to answer, such as "Will the fourth-year Global Health elective allow me to travel to an area on the State Department no travel list?" or "Do you think Dr. Beech will let me join his neurobiology lab?" Again, either ask a question that flows naturally from the previous conversation or that gives the interviewer a chance to show off a bit.

If you have already received interview invites, prepare three questions for each school's potential interviewers now. Repeat this exercise for every interview you will attend. It is unlikely you'll use all three questions, but it will be nice to have them ready just in case.

Chapter 30

Style Prep

Now that you are ready to wow the interviewers with your preparation and poise, we need to talk about your style. I know, after thinking about your biggest mistake and debating who should be the recipient of a new heart, considering your wardrobe seems a bit silly. But how we present ourselves tells others a lot about us. You don't need to be a supermodel, but you do need to look professional.

The Suit

The suit is the medical school interview wardrobe staple. First off, your interview suit needs to fit. Try on your suit, look in the mirror, and ask yourself these questions:

- Does the suit fit?
- Is it too baggy in places?
- Too tight in others?
- Are the sleeves or pants too long or short?
- Is it comfortable to walk and sit?
- Does the suit still look good when I walk and sit?
- Am I repeatedly pulling at my collar, sleeves, or skirt?
- How do I feel?

You don't have to spend hundreds of dollars on a new suit. But you do need a suit that fits, is comfortable, and makes you feel confident. If you have an old suit, take it to a tailor and ensure it fits. If you plan to buy a new suit, spend some time picking the right one and spend the money to have it tailored. Many suit shops will tailor a suit for you as part of the cost. A well-fitted suit is an important item of any professional wardrobe. Make the investment now and you should be able to use the suit for years to come. Remember, suit tailoring changes with the style of the times. In our hipster era, short, tight pants are all the rage. When tailoring your suit, take the long view. A more conservative cut will serve you well for longer.

Second, you don't need to look like you are going to a funeral. I shake my head every time I see medical school interviewees parading through the hospital halls in their dour suits. They look so sad! I'm not saying you should try to dress like a style icon with no socks, high water slacks, and an eye-catching pocket square. And your favorite short skirt that has to be pulled down every minute should probably be left in the closet. Doctors tend to dress more on the conservative end of the spectrum, but you don't need to look dowdy. Look professional.

As for color, you have a range of choices. Navy blue, black, and gray are the most common suit colors. I wore a gorgeous dark green silk suit that stood out in a good way. It's probably not a great idea to wear a baby blue tux à la *Dumb and Dumber*, but there is no rule saying you have to wear a black suit to a medical school interview.

Ladies: You may feel free to wear a pants suit or a suit jacket and skirt. Thankfully, the style mavens have thrown out the rule that you must wear pantyhose with your skirt. Your mom may freak at the idea of not wearing any sort of hose with a skirt, but I promise it is perfectly acceptable these days.

Finally, it is not only acceptable but expected that you will wear the same suit to every interview. The admissions committees don't compare style notes. Find your best look and wear it over and over.

SHIRT

Gents: Your shirt should be pressed and fit well beneath the suit jacket. Shirts that are too big look frumpy as they crease in odd places. Shirts that are too small cause the buttons to stretch at unusual angles and usually have sleeves that are too short. You don't have to wear a white shirt. Blue, off white, light grey, and even light yellow shirts can work. Check how it looks with the suit and tie.

Ladies: You may wear a traditional collared shirt or a camisole. Be sure the shirt you wear is the appropriate length so it does not un-tuck easily or leave an unseemly bulge when tucked in. Since you won't be wearing a tie, think of your shirt as a way to add a pop of color to the suit. If you have made a bold choice on suit color, then it's likely best to go with a neutral shirt.

TIE

Gents: Your tie pulls the entire outfit together. If you have made a conservative choice with the suit and shirt, be sure to add some color in the tie. Ties can be a great source of conversation, so feel free to be a bit creative (while always looking professional).

Ladies: Fortunately, you don't have to think about this part of your wardrobe.

SHOES

Find comfortable shoes that look great with your suit. You will be walking for hours, often in cold climates (read "ice and snow") during the interview day. If you can't play a basketball game in your formal medical school interview shoes, go find another pair. Black shoes are a good bet for most suits. You can get away with brown in some circumstances, but be sure it works. And ladies, please put the five-inch heels back in the closet. There is nothing more embarrassing than a stilted walk due to impossibly high heel length or a turned ankle on an interview day caused by poorly chosen shoes. Finally, be sure the shoes are shined for each interview. An old business interview secret maintains that shoes are the window to a potential hire's work ethic. Shined, well-kept shoes show a person is detail-oriented and dedicated to an overall polished look. Feel free to scoff, but shoes matter.

JEWELRY

As for jewelry, earrings in men are always a point of controversy. If your earring is an important part of who you are, leave it in. But if you consider it just a piece of jewelry, I would take it out. There are certainly more conservative physicians who don't want to accept an applicant that seems like a "punk." This is incredibly out of date, but your interviewer may come from a time when men wearing earrings was less acceptable. Do you really want to throw away your entire application on a piece of jewelry? If you want to make a statement, make sure you get into medical school first.

Ladies, if you'd like to wear jewelry, feel free to wear some on the interview day. Just don't overd0 it. A simple pendant necklace, stud earrings, watch, and comfortable ring are as far as I'd go. Whatever jewelry you do wear, make sure you don't play with it. If you find yourself twirling a ring or watch or playing with a necklace or earrings during a mock interview, don't wear that particular piece on the interview day.

Body piercings that show (nose ring, tongue ring, eyebrow ring, *etc.*) fall under the same general guidelines as earrings in men. Wear it if it is a huge part of who you are. Lose it for a day if it isn't.

Tattoos are all the rage these days. I suggest keeping tattoos covered for medical school interviews unless you feel they are an immensely important part of you that needs to be expressed.

HAIR

When it comes to hair, the medical school interview season is not the time to experiment with the Mohawk you always wanted. Keep hair clean and simple. If you have long hair (men and women), you do not need to cut it. Just be sure it is clean and out of your face. Many people play with their hair when they are nervous. Devise a hairstyle that looks professional and minimizes the chance you will play with it. If you have a non-traditional hair color (blue, purple, pink, *etc.*), think about how important that specific color is to you. There is no problem with making a statement through style, just be sure it is the statement you want to make at a medical school interview.

MAKE-UP

Given it is the ladies who usually wear make-up, I will address this section to you. The key to professional looking make-up is to appear like you aren't wearing make-up! It's better to underdo than overdo. Avoid caking on foundation, applying clumpy mascara, and overdoing eyeliner. If you are someone who never wears make-up, don't feel you need to change for the interview day. But consider a nice shade of lipstick and a touch of blush – they can help create a simple, professional look.

If you are a man who likes to wear make-up, take the approach we have discussed regarding earrings in men, piercings, tattoos, and non-traditional hair color: if you feel wearing make-up is an essential part of who you are, go for it. If not, it's probably best to be make-up free on your medical school interview day.

FIRST 12 INCHES

One of my favorite scribes gave me this style maxim, and I love it for its simplicity: It's the first 12 inches of your head, hands, and feet that matter most.

Head
Keep the cowlick under control
Don't overdo the hair products, make-up, or jewelry
Be clean shaven
Check teeth for errant vegetable matter and lipstick

Hands
Groom nails short and clean
Chipped nail polish is worse than none at all

Feet
Polish your shoes (yes, I actually mean go out and buy real shoe polish and start scrubbing)
For those color-blind guys out there: make sure your socks match
Buy shoes that are comfortable and allow an elegant gait

Etiquette Tips

I am sure these tips will seem obvious, but you would be surprised by the inappropriate behavior of some applicants. I have received e-mails from multiple members of medical school admissions committees requesting I reinforce these principles with pre-meds. Yikes! During an interview, please avoid:

1. Chewing gum
2. Swearing
3. Using racial slurs
4. Speaking in slang
5. Ticking anybody off
6. Saying "like" every sentence

Be as respectful of the administrative assistants as you are of the interviewers. Rude behavior directed toward any of the medical school staff often gets back to the admissions committee and has been known to sink even exceptional candidates.

Further, *any* communication you have with the medical school, be it via phone or e-mail, must be in a formal, professional manner. Address everyone by formal title (*i.e.*, Dr. Miller, Mrs. Brown, *etc.*). Consider e-mails to be more like formal letters than text messages or tweets. Don't use abbreviations or slang. Is this obvious? Yes. Fantastic, then you won't have an etiquette issue.

We've come to the end of the Style Prep chapter. Spend the rest of today planning your interview wardrobe. Make sure you allow enough time to tailor the suit if need be. And consider modeling your outfit to others and receiving feedback before the interview day.

CHAPTER 31

Final Preparation

You have practiced, practiced, and practiced some more, reviewed your application, picked the perfect interview suit, and shined your shoes. Before you leave for an interview, remember these final details:

- If you are flying, pack all clothes in a carry-on. I learned the value of this tip the hard way. I didn't show up in jeans to an important interview but came darn close. Airlines lose baggage frequently. Always carry on your luggage.
- Ensure your toiletries are packed well enough to avoid staining your clothes should leakage occur.
- Bring an extra tie and shirt (for the gents) and shirt (for the ladies) in case a disastrous spill happens.
- Be sure you have all directions, including public transit options, mapped out. Being late to a medical school interview is not an option.
- Bring to the interview a professional-looking bag filled with:
  - A legal pad. Everyone seems to bring a fancy, leather portfolio with a legal pad inside to interviews. But have you ever seen someone actually taking notes? There is no need to take notes during the interview, as that may seem

pretentious. But you can use the portfolio to store some important items and take notes post interview.

- o Store a copy of your AMCAS application, secondary application for the school you are visiting, and any publications/abstracts in the portfolio's inside folder. This will allow you to review these items prior to the interview or during breaks in the interview day. It is unlikely any interviewers will ask to see your publications, but it's not unheard of - so best to be prepared.
- o Put a small roll of dental floss into the pocket as well. I can't tell you how many times I've seen pre-meds with food stuck in their teeth when interviews occur after a meal. Having floss might just save you from an embarrassing situation.
- o Take notes after each interview. Include:
  - Interview date
  - Interviewer's name and title spelled correctly (you may ask for the interviewer's card at the close of the interview)
  - Topics discussed
  - School positives
  - School negatives
  - Overall gut reaction - Taking five minutes to log your thoughts will help you keep the details of each school straight in your mind and remember specifics to put in thank you notes. As schools start to blur together on the interview trail, these notes will be very helpful.
- o Blank thank you notes with envelopes and stamps
- o A snack
- o Your extra shirt/tie
- Ensure a good night's sleep not only the night before, but also the night before the night before the interview. Studies have

shown the night previous to the night before an event is the most important night of sleep for excellent performance in any activity.

I suggest you put the book down now and find/buy a portfolio and blank thank you notes. Then print out your AMCAS, secondary essays, and publications and put them in your portfolio with some dental floss. If you have interviews scheduled, take the time now to research your travel plan detailing how you will get yourself to the medical school on time and in case of inclement weather. Be sure to consider a back-up plan should your first mode of transportation not be available.

CHAPTER 32

Post-Interview Strategy

After an interview, give yourself a pat on the back and get ready, as there is still more work to be done to increase your chances of getting into medical school. Employing a strategic approach to communicating with schools after the interview may help you get in.

Before you contact any medical school, check their communication policy. Some schools allow you to contact them at any time and welcome all communication. Others only want to be contacted post an interview or even not at all. The contact policy is usually posted on the medical school's admissions website. Do not contact a no contact school.

Also pay attention to how schools want to be contacted. Some still want paper. Others prefer e-mail. Still others have an online portal for submitting supplemental information. If there are no details listed on a medical school's website, you may assume they accept any form of contact anytime.

One key to the post-interview strategy is not to overdo it. Medical schools don't want to receive dozens of updates from you or your recommenders. Focus on creating high-impact communication per the strategy laid out below.

There are four main ways to communicate with a school after an interview:

1. Thank you notes
2. Letter of intent/update letters
3. Verbal recommendation
4. Written recommendation

Let's walk through these one-by-one.

Thank You Notes

I suggest you write a handwritten thank you note to every interviewer at any school (that accepts post-interview communication) you might attend if accepted. Thank you notes are an easy way to remind the interviewer of you and your strengths so that she can advocate for you to the admissions committee.

When it is common for an interviewer to receive hundreds of e-mails a day, why send such an important communication to an already full e-mail inbox? Yes, handwriting thank you notes is old school. But it's effective. Here are some tricks to make writing these letters easy and efficient:

1. Bring thank you notes, envelopes, and stamps with you to the interview.
2. After every interview, note the interviewer's name and title and three things you discussed that led to an engaging conversation.
3. Immediately after you finish the interview(s), head to a coffee shop to debrief and relax. Write the thank you notes and drop them in a mailbox that day. Of course, you can write the notes on your way home on the plane, train, *etc.*, but delaying thank you notes until "later" often means you will never write them.

4. Given many rolling admissions schools meet to discuss your application within days of the interview, you want to get these thank you notes in the mail as soon as possible.

You can use the same formula for every thank you note. Here's an example:

> "Dear Dr. Miller,
> It was a pleasure to meet you on December 17 and hear about Man's Greatest Medical School's new curriculum aligning system-based learning with early clinical rotations and cutting-edge research opportunities. I especially appreciated your interest in my recent study on marathon running and its effect on cardiovascular health and will update you when the manuscript is accepted for publication. I also enjoyed talking about the recent success of the DC University basketball team, and I hope you will see us in the NCAA tournament again this year. Have a wonderful holiday.
> Sincerely,
> Jane Doe"

As you can see in this thank you note example, you want to:

- Spell the interviewer's name correctly and use the appropriate prefix
- Remind the interviewer of the interview date
- Express specific interest in the school in areas such as:
  - Curriculum
  - Research
  - Community service
  - Extracurricular activities
  - Clinical opportunities

- o Population served
- o Location
- Highlight your strengths and unique characteristics discussed in the interview in areas such as:
- o Research
- o Community service
- o Athletics/arts/extracurriculars
- o Clinical experience
- Close with a cordial statement

Here's another thank you note example:

"Dear Dr. Bruno,

Thank you for taking time out of your practice to interview me on February 4. I enjoyed discussing how your clinical research on diabetes aligns with what I have been exploring in Dr. Mann's Laboratory. Did you see the recent paper in *Cell* on the novel transmitter found? I think you'll find it very interesting. I've also been thinking about the conversation we had about the Affordable Care Act's hidden successes and how doctors must all play a role in policy. Inspired, I plan to join the health policy club at school and look forward to reading on these subjects more deeply. I very much enjoyed my time at South University and thank you for supporting my application.

Kind regards,

Jim Baily"

This thank you note does a few things very well:

- Engaging the reader by asking a question about a recent paper relevant to the interview discussion and showing the author continues to be involved in medical research topics

- Giving specifics about joining the policy club shows the author is curious and well-suited to a profession requiring life-long learning
- By ending with "thank you for supporting my application," the author is reminding the interviewer in a subtle and polite way that the interviewer does play a large role in whether or not he gains acceptance

Thank you notes are not hard, but they can be tedious. Use these examples as a format and get your letters done as soon as you can after the actual interviews.

LETTER OF INTENT/UPDATE LETTERS

A helpful thing to remember in medical school admissions is that schools want to be wanted. Some schools will come out and say it, requesting you send a letter of intent if the school is your top choice. Other schools tend to be coy about it, but they still want to be wanted. In fact, medical schools collect statistics on their acceptance rate and use it as one measure of success. Therefore, telling a school you will attend if accepted is powerful tool you may use to increase your chances of acceptance.

Of course, you may only tell one school it is your top choice. Even if this decision changes over time, I believe it is unethical to send letters of intent to two schools. The only caveat to this is if you have sent a letter of intent to a school and been rejected. It is then acceptable to choose another top choice and send a letter to it. Update letters, on the other hand, may be sent to multiple schools. The only real difference between a letter of intent and an update letter is that a letter of intent states the school is your top choice, while an update letter does not. I suggest sending a letter of intent as soon as you know a school is your top choice. This tends to happen after the interview. Update letters are a bit more flexible. They are most often sent in an attempt to get off a hold/waitlist. However, update letters can be used to gain an interview if it is late in the season or to increase your chances of acceptances at schools you have not heard from post interview.

Here are some tips on writing a letter of intent/update letter:

- Use a formal tone
- Keep to less than one page (can be single spaced)
- Send via regular mail and e-mail (if schools allows all types of communication)
- Include a formal letter opening with your address, date, recipient address, and salutation in the letter sent via regular mail. Only the salutation is required for the e-mail.
- Use the following structure:

Address to dean of admissions
(e.g., "Dear Dean Brown,")

Paragraph I
Open with your reason for writing. If writing a letter of intent, be sure to state the school is your top choice and you would attend if accepted.

Paragraph II
Provide update(s) if any exist.

Paragraph III
Discuss why you are a good fit for the school. Be specific. You can merge paragraphs II and III if your updates lend themselves to explaining why you are a good fit for the school.

Paragraph IV

Discuss reasons the school is a good fit for you. Again, be specific. (Paragraphs III and IV can be flipped if desired)

Closing

Finish with a formal closing, also known as a complementary close (*e.g.*, "Sincerely"), your signature with typed name beneath, and AMCAS ID.

A few examples will help you see how to write a letter of intent/ update letter. Please note, these letters were all written by pre-meds who gained acceptance to medical school. Thus, I have removed or modified all identifying items from these letters to maintain privacy. In your letters, of course, you want to include date, address, and real names of schools/programs/places, *etc.*

Example 1: Letter of Intent

This example is a letter of intent because if states "your university is my first choice for medical school, and I will attend if accepted." It follows the structure outlined above but flips the third and fourth paragraph: Dear Dean [last name of dean of admissions] → Opening with reason for writing → Update → Why school is good fit for you with specifics → Why you are a good fit for school with specifics → Complementary close and signature with typed name and AMCAS ID. The version being sent by regular mail should also include a formal letter opening with your address, date, and the recipient's address.

The letter example below is a tad long, but it does put forth a good argument for why this student should be accepted. Again, remember I have removed all identifiers from this example. When you write a letter, use the formal names. For example, instead of the generic, "inpatients at a tertiary academic center" in the example letter, use the real name of the tertiary academic center in your letter.

"Dear Dean Martin,

After interviewing last week, I am confident your university is my first choice for medical school, and I will attend if accepted.

Since submitting my application, I have expanded my role as a research study coordinator within the Medicine Division at University School of Medicine. Two projects have been selected for an abstract presentation at an international research conference. Given this success, I am working to publish a first author manuscript in the next several months.

During my interview, I confirmed your school aligns with what I seek in a medical school – holistic medical education, diversity of academic opportunities, and a strong support network. It was a pleasure speaking with Dr. Wharton about how his experience as a medical student prepared him to be a well-rounded clinician and discussing the support students receive to pursue individual interests. I look forward to personalizing my medical education through the track options and continuing research to prevent racial and gender disparities in medicine. Further, my student interviewer informed me how I can continue collaborating with peers, working with diverse and Spanish-speaking patient populations, and helping underserved communities through participation in the Student Group and Urban Clinic.

As a non-traditional applicant, I bring a unique background and experience with diverse patient populations and practice settings. Working and volunteering with patients in a surgery clinic, indigent immigrants in a community clinic, and inpatients at a tertiary academic center, I have confirmed the imperative of teamwork to success and the important role of culture in medicine. My penchant for collaboration and cultural sensitivity fits in well with your school's focus on creating a supportive environment, early clinical experience, and cultural competency.

Your school's community will undoubtedly provide me with the ideal environment to grow into a primary care physician who delivers culturally-sensitive care to disadvantaged populations. Thank you for your time and consideration. Sincerely,

Jamie Smith
AMCAS ID: 00000001"

Example 2: Letter of Intent

This example is also a letter of intent because of the line "MGMS is my top choice for medical school, and I would attend if accepted." The letter varies slightly from example 1 because it merges the update paragraph with the why-you-are-a-good-fit-for-the-school paragraph. Here is the structure: Dear Dean [last name of dean of admissions] → Opening with reason for writing → Update merged with why you are a good fit for school → Why school is a good fit for you with specifics → Complementary close and signature with typed name and AMCAS ID. Please again note, all identifiers in this letter have been removed or modified to maintain privacy.

"Dear Dean Smith,

I am writing with the goal of obtaining acceptance into the Man's Greatest Medical School Class of 2021 and updating you on my recent activities. Interviewing on November 5 confirmed that MGMS is my top choice for medical school, and I would attend if accepted.

Since November, I have completed two advanced science courses in physiology and anatomy, earning an A in each. I have also taken a medical Spanish immersion course and look forward to continuing to improve my language skills through MGMS's Service for Latin America missions and by volunteering at the Somos Hermanos free clinic. I have also continued my work as a clinical research assistant at University Hospital and have been invited to speak at an international conference in Zurich on my findings regarding the treatment of congestive heart failure. The Center for Integrated Cardiac Care at MGMS will certainly provide an excellent place for me to continue my research.

Given its focus on teaching, emphasis on serving disadvantaged populations, and location, MGMS is the ideal place for me to continue my journey to becoming a doctor. Having spent over 100 hours shadowing in an academic center, I have seen the positive impact a culture of teaching can have on trainees of every level. As a teaching assistant for the last three years, I am passionate about entering an environment where we all learn from each other. Further, my service to underprivileged communities as president of my university's chapter of Unite for Sight has shown me how poverty negatively impacts health. My values align with MGMS's core mission to serve those who need the most help. Finally, I am a native Montanan and am passionate about both staying in my home state and assisting the community I have been a part of since birth.

I believe my academic ability, research creativity, interest in teaching, and passion for serving the disadvantaged of Montana will make me an asset to MGMS. Thank you for taking the time to review my application.

Sincerely,

Bob Jones
AMCAS ID: 00000002"

Example 3: Update Letter

The following letter is an update letter (not a letter of intent) because it does not say the applicant would attend if accepted. But notice how the language still makes a strong case for the author's interest in the school. In reality, the difference between a letter of intent and an update letter may be one sentence. Also notice how the author makes clear where she stands – she has been placed on hold. Stating this allows her to make the goal clear without saying she would attend if accepted.

This author takes a different structural approach to the letter. She provides three updates (one per paragraph) and links each one to the school of interest. Feel free to use this structure should you also have this many impressive updates. Once again, all identifiers in this letter have been removed or modified to maintain privacy.

> "Dear Dr. Cook,
>
> After interviewing at North Medical School at the end of October, I received a hold from the admissions committee but have yet to be notified of a final decision. I am particularly interested in NMS and am writing to update you on my activities in hope the information can assist in making your admissions decision.
>
> In November, I started a full-time position working on the general medical/surgical unit of the local hospital. This unit serves mostly oncology patients with an emphasis on end-of-life care. In addition to learning how these cases are managed after admission, I have become interested in the ethical decisions surrounding palliative care. While numerous recent newspaper articles have discussed medical ethics as a result of the national healthcare debate, I have found the concrete examples occurring everyday on the unit complex and compelling. The decisions that must be made by patients and their families are

always more nuanced than the typical media portrayal. I am further developing my own ethical beliefs and learning how best to shape interactions with families to help them through difficult end-of-life decisions. I expect the ethics course offered as an elective during NMS's second-year curriculum will help me continue to inform my stance on biomedical ethics topics.

I am also volunteering one full day a week in the medical operations department of an international medical aid organization. I am excited about the organization's work building international friendships through medicine and focusing on improved health care in the developing world by training health care workers in those countries. I hope to continue volunteering with this impressive organization throughout medical school.

Finally, I have retaken the MCAT, scoring in the 95th percentile. Along with my strong GPA in the notoriously challenging field of engineering, I believe this score provides more evidence of my ability to excel in the academically rigorous medical school environment.

I look forward to hearing from your office soon and greatly appreciate your consideration and careful review.

Sincerely,

Maya Morton
AMCAS ID: 00000003"

VERBAL RECOMMENDATION

You've completed your thank you notes, written an outstanding letter of intent, and composed update letters to at least your next top five schools. Now what? Most of the time, that will be enough. But if you find yourself vying for a spot in an incredibly competitive school, stuck on waitlists, or trying to gain an interview late in the application season, you may consider asking someone to make a verbal recommendation on your behalf. This can be either a recommender who already wrote a letter or someone new. If the person happens to have an affiliation with the school, all the better. But this is not essential.

The call should come only from a recommender who knows you well. A call from your uncle's cousin's wife who has met you once but happened to graduate from your waitlisted school will not be of much help and might even hurt you. So be smart. Start with your college's pre-med advisor and see if he will make a call on your behalf. The answer is often no, but it's worth a shot. If that doesn't work out, think of your biggest champion or mentor (who is not related to you) and ask her to call. You only need one person to make the call.

I'm often asked, "Whom should the recommender call and what should he say?" The answer is – it depends. The recommender needs to be comfortable playing it by ear. He should try to call the dean of admissions. If that contact is difficult to make, anyone on the admissions committee will do. Once someone with the power to make an admissions decision is on the line, the recommender can spend a few minutes making the case for your acceptance. This can be something very simple, such as "Hi, I'm Dr. Miller, and I am calling on behalf of John Doe. I've worked with him in the emergency department for the last two years and have only exceptional things to say. I wanted to call because I hear he is waitlisted and think you should give his application another good look. He has the talent, people skills, and determination required to be an excellent physician." These conversations often continue naturally for a few minutes. But even if the call is short, the recommender just got your name in front of someone on the admissions committee. Sometimes "another good look" is all you need to gain acceptance.

I suggest only one call per school and one call per recommender. In general, you will use this tactic for your top school. If you are fortunate to have multiple people willing to make calls for you, then you can have different recommenders call different schools. Verbal recommendations are not required to get in, and they really should be used sparingly. There are many instances where pre-meds can't find the right person to make the call. No worries! If a verbal recommendation doesn't work out, consider obtaining an additional written recommendation as per the next section.

WRITTEN RECOMMENDATION

You may have a recommender, hopefully someone different than the verbal recommender, write an additional formal letter of evaluation for you. As with any recommendation, you want the person who writes the letter to know you well and to provide a glowing reference. Use this letter to highlight your strengths, show you have improved a hole in your application, provide evidence of your well roundedness, or update the admissions committee on a recent accomplishment. If you haven't read it already, pick up *The Medical School Admissions Guide* and review the section on recommendations where you will learn exactly how to ask for a written recommendation. There is a system and it is important to ask for a written recommendation correctly.

Unlike a verbal recommendation, where one person calls one school, you may send the written recommendation to any schools where you haven't been rejected and that accept communications beyond the primary and secondary applications. Remember to check the contact policy of every school. The easiest way to send an additional recommendation is to use a service like Interfolio that allows the recommender to upload the letter to a secure server and you to then transmit the letter to individual schools. Please note, these services charge a fee. Of course, some schools require you to communicate in a particular manner, such as submitting extra material via e-mail or through the school's intranet. But you know this because you've already checked each school's communication policy, right?

Don't overdo it on the additional recommendations. I suggest one phone call and one written recommendation to any one school at most. Annoying the admissions staff with excessive communication rarely leads to a good outcome.

Let's review the post-interview strategy timeline:

Communication	Person	Timeline
Thank you notes	Individual interviewer	Immediately post interview
Letter of intent	Dean of admissions	Post interview Once top choice identified
Update letters	Dean of admissions	Usually post interview When update available Often when on hold/ waitlist May send to request interview
Verbal recommendation	Dean of admissions OR Ad com member	Usually post interview Once top choice identified May use to request interview

Communication	Person	Timeline
Written recommendation	Dean of admissions	Usually post interview May send to multiple schools May use to request interview

If you had to decide right now, whom would you ask for verbal and written recommendations? If no one comes to mind, take the time to brainstorm a list of potential verbal and written recommenders.

Congratulations! We've reached the end of our medical school interview preparation discussion. Though it may initially feel overwhelming, you now have an excellent strategy for approaching the before, during, and after of medical school interviews. If you haven't already, schedule at least one mock interview with your pre-med committee and/or an admissions consultant. I have found most pre-meds benefit from two and sometimes three mock interviews. I've rarely seen a pre-med improve much after three mock interviews and sometimes receiving feedback from too many different sources can be confusing. So plan accordingly. I do hope you found this book helpful and wish you the best of luck as you pursue your dreams!

For more tips on gaining interviews late in the game and preparing for DO/Caribbean school interviews, flip forward to the appendices.

APPENDIX A

No Interviews Yet. Now What?

Let's assume it's December or January of your application year and you haven't received any interviews. Though it is late in the game, there are a few things you can do to determine if there is a problem with your application requiring immediate action:

1. Review your AMCAS and secondary applications with a medical school expert, such as your school's pre-med advisor or a medical school admissions consultant. I recently had a client who realized certain classes had been categorized incorrectly on the AMCAS application, making the science GPA inappropriately low. This kind of issue can sink a medical school application and needs to be addressed immediately through the appropriate AMCAS channels, such as submitting an official academic request form.

2. Create a spreadsheet to organize where you stand. List school name, date of secondary application receipt, date of secondary application submission, and whether you received an e-mail confirmation stating the application is complete. If you did not receive a confirmation e-mail, call the school's admissions office and ask if your application is complete and if all interview invites have been given. You may find a secondary you submitted was never received. You will also learn if some interview invites remain.

3. Call each school where you have applied but have not received a secondary and ensure the school has everything it needs prior to sending a secondary application. Also inquire about whether any more secondaries will be sent out (quite unlikely at this stage in the medical school cycle, but it doesn't hurt to ask).

The key here is to look for help and ask questions. Ignoring the situation because you are too busy or afraid of the answers is not the way to go. Get informed and fix any errors. You never know, asking for expert advice and making a few phone calls to medical schools could mean the difference between medical school acceptance and rejection.

If you are one of the lucky ones who have received many interviews and perhaps acceptances, consider canceling interviews at schools you would not attend if accepted. The medical school interview trail can be exhausting. Think about canceling some of the interviews to avoid burnout. For example, you have already been accepted to one of your top choices and have a few "safety school" interviews in February. Do yourself and the admissions committees a favor and call to cancel those interviews. Also think of those who have not yet received interviews. Your cancellation may open a spot for another applicant. There are no awards given to those who receive the most medical school interviews or admissions offers.

APPENDIX B

Osteopathic (DO) School Interviews

Though osteopathic (DO) schools have a completely separate application (AACOMAS) from allopathic schools (AMCAS), the interviews tend to be very similar to "traditional" medical school interviews. Just like MD schools, DO institutions employ one-on-one and group interviews and use open, semi-open, or closed file. Interestingly, group interviews tend to be more common for DO than MD schools.

What you have already read in this book will prepare you well for DO interviews. However, there are some DO-specific questions that require your attention. I can almost guarantee you will be asked one or more of the following questions:

1. Why DO?
2. What specifically do you like most about osteopathic medicine?
3. How many osteopathic physicians have you shadowed/observed?
4. Are you applying to allopathic schools as well?
5. Have you applied before?

When preparing responses, remember osteopathic schools often are made to feel like second-class citizens when compared to allopathic schools. Everyone knows DO admissions are less competitive than

MD, and the majority of DO applicants would rather go to an allopathic medical school if they could gain acceptance. The DO admissions committees can't stand this! They want applicants who want to be DOs, as opposed to candidates with holes in their application or pre-meds looking for a safety school. When preparing for DO interviews, be sure you understand the history and underlying philosophy of osteopathic medicine so you can prove why you want to be a DO, as opposed to why you couldn't become a MD.

Let's walk through these questions one by one.

DO Q1: *Why DO?*

DO A1: "Because of my MCAT score [or GPA or institutional action or lack of research, *etc.*]" is not an appropriate answer. Head back to Chapter 6 and review your answers to the motivation for medicine queries. You don't need a whole new response for DO schools. You just need to connect your answer to the values of osteopathy – holism, prevention, and the benefit of training in manipulation (chiropractic) techniques. You could adapt your response by beginning with a statement that shows you understand what a DO is all about. For example, "I am drawn to the core values of osteopathy, such as treating the whole patient and focusing on preventative medicine." Then you can move into your prepared motivation for medicine answer, ensuring each part connects back in some way to osteopathic medicine's core tenets.

DO Q2: *What specifically do you like most about osteopathic medicine?*

DO A2: This question is really asking, "Do you know what osteopathic medicine is all about, or are you applying here because your application is not competitive enough for allopathic schools?" Prove to the interviewer your interest in osteopathic medicine by discussing its core values, which you have already reviewed for DO Q1. As you already know by now, it is best to connect your answer to a personal experience. For example,

"My favorite part of osteopathic medicine is the focus on holistic medicine. While volunteering at a free clinic in downtown Detroit, I saw how poverty directly affected every aspect of patients' lives, including their health. It was like dominos. Poverty led to poor food choices that led to obesity that led to diabetes. I want to train to become the kind of physician who understands how every aspect of patient's history – social, economic, cultural, mental, and physical – affects his or her health, and then use this understanding to provide comprehensive treatment. Osteopathic medicine is the best place to obtain this kind of holistically-focused training."

DO Q3: *How many osteopathic physicians have you shadowed/observed?*

DO A3: Given the DO application strongly suggests you have a DO "sponsor," I know you have at least one person you can discuss. The point of this question is similar to that of the previous two queries: to ensure you have done your homework and understand the intricacies of osteopathic medicine. If your interview is in a few weeks and you don't have a good answer to this question, go shadow some more DO physicians! Further, instead of giving only a number, provide some specifics:

"I have shadowed three DO physicians – Dr. Miller in emergency medicine, Dr. Green in internal medicine/primary care, and Dr. Smith in anesthesiology. It was inspiring to see how three physicians utilized the DO path to enter their first-choice specialties."

DO Q4: *Are you applying to allopathic schools as well?*

DO A4: Be honest and answer, "Yes" or, "No," and then be ready to explain why. Even if you are applying DO because your application is not competitive for allopathic schools, prepare a response that has a positive tone and speaks well of the DO degree. Further, don't feel like you have to apologize for applying to both. You can simply state you are casting a wide net to maximize your options.

DO Q5: *Have you applied before?*

DO A5: DO interviewers often ask this question because many DO applicants have already applied once to allopathic schools and are using DO as a "back-up." Take the same tactic as in DO Q4 – be honest, stay positive, and don't apologize.

Here's the bottom line for DO interviews: be ready to speak about *why* you want to obtain a DO degree as opposed to the more traditional MD. And be able to make this case without emphasizing your negatives or bad-talking allopathic schools. Keep it positive.

APPENDIX C

Caribbean School Interviews

Caribbean medical school interviews are very similar to US-based MD and DO interviews. They tend to be one-on-one, open file interviews with one to three admissions committee members or students. Some schools ask you to write an essay (St. George is known for this) before or after the interviews. What's unique about Caribbean interviews is that they often take place in a regional location, as opposed to at the actual school. This is a convenience, but it does not allow you to get a vibe for the school in person. If you are applying to Caribbean schools, I highly suggest you visit the campus and speak with current students prior to making your final decision on where to attend medical school. Caribbean medical schools do not expect you to fly to visit the school prior to the interview, but they do want you to have done research on the school and to have thought about how you will handle going to school off the mainland.

Other than the interview questions already addressed in this book, Caribbean medical schools tend to ask two other types of questions:

C Q1: *Why Caribbean (as opposed to US-based MD or DO)?*

C A1: Every interviewer will ask some form of this question. Sometimes the interviewer will ask, "Why do you want to attend [name of school]?" or "Did you apply to any US medical schools or receive interviews?" These queries are probing your motivation for applying to a non-traditional type of school. As